The Triangle of Health: Mental/Emotional Components

On The Inside Press

Ojai, CA

To all my friends and relatives

Thank you for your love, kindness, and support.

The Triangle of Health: Mental/Emotional Components

DR. VLADIMIR GORDIN

Published by **On The Inside Press**

Every effort has been made to ensure that the information contained within this publication is accurate at the time of printing. However, this book is not an attempt by the author to render medical services to the individual reader, and should not be taken as such. This publication presents only the author's opinions, based upon his knowledge, experience and beliefs. This book is not intended to be, and must not be taken as, a replacement for consulting with your healthcare provider. Consult with a qualified healthcare provider if you are injured, or if you suffer from any medical condition. The author or publisher shall in no way be held liable or responsible for any loss or damage allegedly arising from any information contained within this book.

Author: Dr. Vladimir Gordin

Phone: (847) 243-2110

Email: info@gordinmedical.com

Websites:

www.GordinMedical.com

www.HealMeVladimir.com

www.Health1240.com

Book Design:

Writers for the Future, LLC.

Email: Writers.for.the.Future@gmail.com

Web: FutureWrit.com, AlexanderPhoenix.com

A complete listing of picture credits can be found at the back of this book.

ISBN 978-0-9882652-1-9

Table of Content

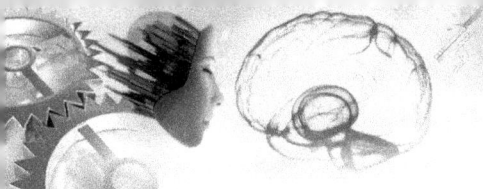

Chapter 1:

The Triangle of Health

The triangle of health is a map depicting the relationships between the structural, chemical, and mental/emotional elements of health and their functions. Our bodies are harmoniously aligned when all the elements work together properly. The structural element includes not only our bones, joints and muscles but also includes the various activities of life such as exercise, rest and physical work (Health Triangle, 2012). The chemical element includes major organs, body chemistry, physiology, hormones, regulatory systems, and the immune system but also refers to diet and nutrition. The mental/emotional element involves some of the most treasured elements of our beings, including our feelings, thoughts, memories and spiritual beliefs.

Aspects of the Triangle of Health:

Structural

Our bodies experience natural traumas in the course of our lives. Childbirth is one of the first such major traumas that our bodies go through; albeit one of the natural processes of life. Additionally, accidents and falls can occur at any time in the course of our lives and injuries can also occur while playing sports. If such an injury is severe, it can significantly interfere with one's quality of life.

Inevitably, the mental/emotional and chemical aspects also affect the physical side of the triangle of health. When the structural aspect is weakened, additional mental and emotional stresses can come to interfere with the natural balance of our being.

Maintaining physical health is much more important than one might think. Physical health is managed by our physical activity, a proper diet, stable mental/emotional health, and the proper usage of nutritional or dietary supplements. One's health suffers when one or more of these elements are interrupted or interfered with. The basic idea here is that maintaining a balance within the body's triangle keeps our body working like a well-oiled machine.

If an injury occurs, we depend upon the body to repair it. The injury must be corrected in the same physical or emotional manner in which the injury occurred. If we put impurities into our bodies and a subsequent accident or injuries were to take place, the healing process should begin by ceasing the intake of such impurities. Another factor in maintaining proper physical health is staying at a healthy weight, which adds to the overall harmony of the body and keeps all aspects of our physical structures sound.

Treatments for maintaining physical health include acupuncture, Applied Kinesiology, massage therapy, chiropractic care and cranial-sacral therapies. These treatments help our bones, joints, muscles, nerves and organs. Nutritional, dietary, herbal, or whole food supplements can also help to maintain our bone, nerve, joint and muscle health.

Mental/Emotional

Mental health is determined by our ability to handle and manage stress in our everyday lives. We cannot always control

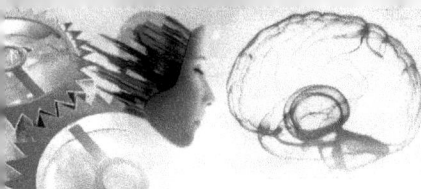

the situations that we experience in life but can certainly play a part in their outcome.

Using healthy strategies to solve problems and manage stress will help keep our mental and emotional balance stable. The general idea is to retain an optimistic outlook on life.

One of the largest strains on our mental and emotional health is personal relationships, particularly, the relationships that we have with our friends and family. These can often cause tension or emotional distress that can in turn affect our peace of mind. Even old emotional distress can affect the emotional side the triangle. Events from our past frequently remind us of painful times in our lives and can lead to temporary emotional breakdowns. A divorce from years past, especially when children have been involved is a prime example. Nevertheless, we sometimes assume that we've dealt with an emotionally traumatic situation completely only to later discover that there were parts of it still retained in our minds.

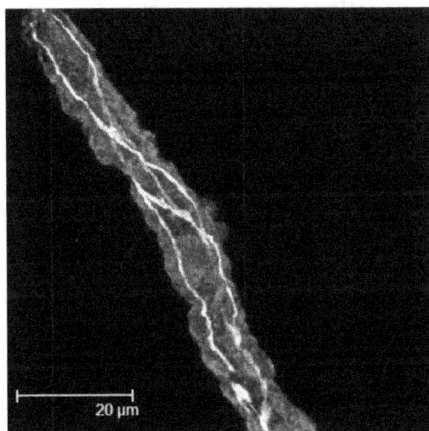

A micro-vessel within the brain

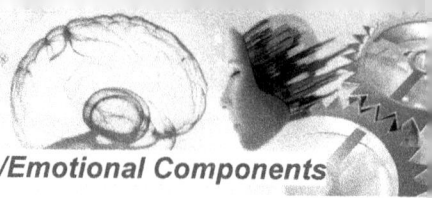

Our brains communicate with our bodies both consciously and unconsciously. When the two do not connect, our natural harmony is disrupted. An upheaval of our emotions can result in both mental stress and physical stress. Our minds and emotions can affect how we feel physically. Emotional stress can be reflected in our self esteem, posture or body language. We often wear our hearts on our sleeves without realizing it. It has been inarguably proven that our minds can cause physical illness. For instance, a person who suffers from worry frequently can develop hives on his or her body. Likewise, a person experiencing emotional stress can develop backaches and headaches. The health of the entire body can be thrown out of balance if one part of the triangle of health is stressed. The chemical side of the triangle can also be affected by mental or emotional distress. For example, our metabolisms can slow down from increased mental stress.

Learning how to manage our mental health may seem like an impossible task. It is up to us to rearrange our thought processes and reactions to reduce the mental stress that we experience in handling different incidents in our daily lives, as well as the unforeseen. The learning process helps us develop skills, knowledge and behaviors to enable us to better ourselves. This process increases our ability to analyze a situation and control how we react to it, whereas not learning healthy problem-solving skills can put us at risk for anxiety disorders or depression. Mental illnesses that are associated with mental distress or emotional trouble include Bipolar Disorder, Depression, Schizophrenia, and various phobias.

Severe emotional distress can cause us to revert to an unhealthy lifestyle and negative thought processes. One can feel defeated, or feel as if there were no options available to climb out of a rut of overwhelming emotion. It has been

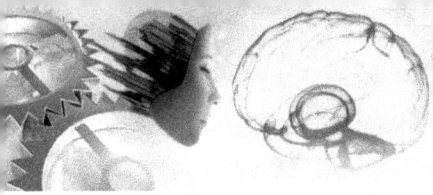

recognized that a therapist or psychologist can only do so much for us in this aspect of our lives.

Therapy sessions can last for years and still not yield positive results. This is often because we're not using the full power of our own minds to work through things: we're using methods instilled into us by another. Those methods may not actually be healthy for us and may cause us to relive our thoughts for a longer period of time than we are comfortable with. We all have the strength within us to decipher a healthy thought process, and to handle mental and emotional stresses with positive results.

It is, ultimately, up to us to clear the emotional stresses from our lives in a healthy way by ensuring that each situation that we encounter experiences closure. The more aware we become regarding to our mental and emotional triggers, the better we can handle each situation as it arises. While tools can be given to us by a professional, it is up to each individual to use those tools properly to maintain stable emotional health.

Chemical

Substances that we put in our bodies can have a negative effect on the chemical side of the triangle.

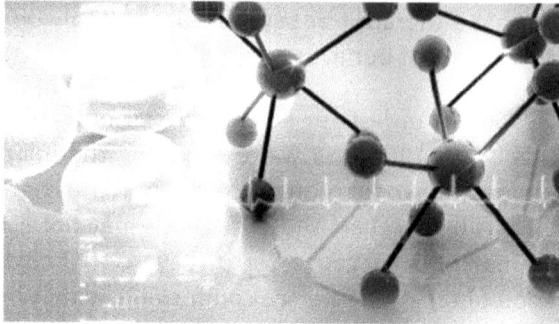

Substances such as nicotine, caffeine, alcohol and narcotics interrupt our body's natural harmony and balance. Not maintaining a healthy, balanced diet can also throw off the triangle. When our bodies do not receive proper nutrition, this can negatively affect our organs and overall body function. Our organs become tired, making it harder for them to sustain the natural functions of the body. When we are fatigued or physically strained, we become more emotionally vulnerable and sensitive. It makes us less capable of handling daily stresses in life. The best way to alleviate or lessen chemical imbalances in the body is to reduce or cease the intake of impure foods and toxins. A detox regimen, under the guidance of a qualified healthcare professional, can also help cleanse our bodies of harmful toxins produced by unhealthy foods, alcohol, drugs and other chemicals (The Triad of Health, 2012).

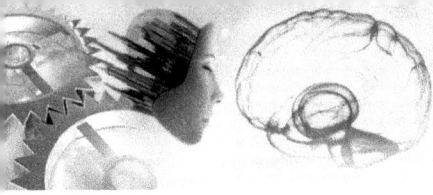

Prefrontal cortex

Medial prefrontal cortex

Ventromedial prefrontal cortex

Amygdala

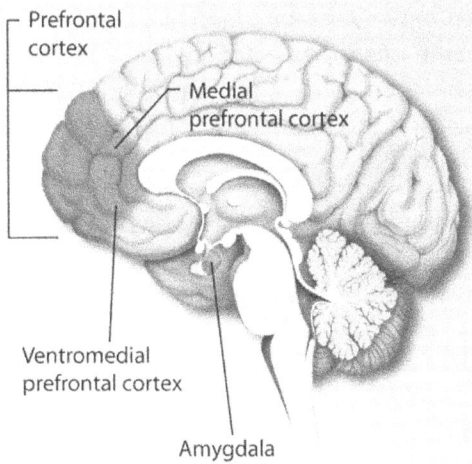

Various areas of the brain

We control what we put into our bodies, and whether or not we're eating right. Similarly, only we can decide to stop smoking, taking illicit drugs or drinking alcohol, along with eliminating or reducing our intake of processed, fatty and sugary foods. We are also responsible for deciding what positive foods to introduce back into our diets. These methods include the use of Applied Kinesiology to improve our range of choices.

Discussing the suggested changes in diet with a highly trained healthcare professional that specializes in natural diets can be helpful. There are some food items that some may not consider to be natural. A highly trained healthcare professional can help determine exactly what is lacking in your diet and what supplements or vitamins should be added to your diet to promote overall health.

Following a natural diet does not necessarily mean always shopping at an organic or health food store. All of the items

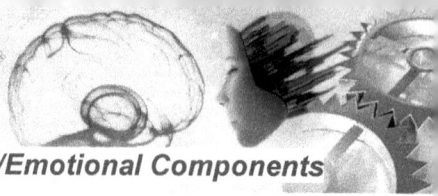

needed to eat healthy can be found in a regular grocery store. It is best to bear in mind that shopping inside the aisles can tempt you to purchase an item that may not be completely pure. Preservatives and additives are an integral part of most prepackaged foods.

These items can build up negative toxins within your brain that may interfere with your mental and emotional health, causing an unwanted additional imbalance in the triangle of health.

Applied Kinesiology practices and trials have developed different techniques in what are known as, 'Specialized Kinesiologies'. The different elements of Specialized Kinesiologies may take on the detection and correction of emotional faults, with others tackling physical or chemical aspects. Using Specialized Kinesiologies removes the need to apply multiple treatments to the same issues. It is important to understand how Specialized Kinesiologies and Applied Kinesiology work in order to move forward in understanding the rest of the triangle of health.

When the right type of treatment is applied, a problem rarely reoccurs or even remains a factor governing your health. The only thing that could bring back an old issue or reverse such progress would be a new trauma. This new trauma can be similar or completely different but can have the same detrimental effect on the psyche.

Applied Kinesiology and the Triangle of Health

During the 1970's, an eminent Chiropractor, George Goodheart, observed that most of our muscles are connected to a specific organ or gland. His determination came from testing muscles

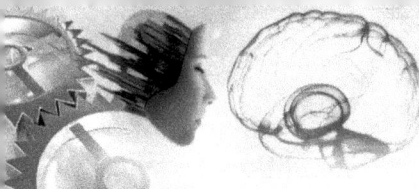

and their weaknesses or strengths. With these observations, he could determine whether a problem was within a muscle or specifically within an organ or gland. He isolated a weak muscle and found that most muscle weaknesses can be corrected with the addition of vitamins, minerals and other supplements. This original technique of Applied Kinesiology paved the way for other techniques savvy readers might know of such as TBM (Total Body Modification), NET (Neuro Emotional Technique), EFT (Emotional Freedom Technique), NRT (Nutrition Response Testing), Callahan and many others. TBM was developed by Dr. Victor Frank. NET was developed by Dr. Scott Walker. The difference between all these techniques and how they are used is beyond the scope of this book.

Applied Kinesiology has developed by leaps and bounds since Dr. Goodheart's original work and is sometimes called Autonomic Reflex Testing, among other names Expensive treatments and invasive procedures are no longer needed to diagnose and treat many problems and issues. In traditional medicine, 'normal' is determined by the examination of several people with and without certain complaints. As a result, traditional medicine generally doesn't take a person's individual situation into consideration in making a decision or determination.

In contract to traditional medicine, Applied Kinesiology takes the whole individual into consideration. These processes have been used for well over 40 years and have been tested on thousands of patients to determine that the techniques work and are beneficial. In many cases, Applied Kinesiology is actually the quickest method to use in order to sort out the complexities of health issues, and to determine an appropriate course of action.

This process is a system of healing that uses muscle testing to gain information from multiple levels in our bodies. Muscles are tested by activating the muscle stress reflex with patients holding specific positions to determine the amount of weakness within a muscle or muscle group. This is also paired with testing tendon reflexes... Since the brain's pain signals regarding a hurt muscle forces us to want to relax or stop an action (to protect the weak muscle), errors due to mental states can be dismissed.

Applied Kinesiology can be, and is, used to diagnose and correct muscle weakness, imbalances and atrophy; most commonly it is used in sports medicine by trainers and athletes. One of the most amazing things about Applied Kinesiology is the fact that it can help obtain information about internal organs, nutritional health and various emotional issues. Stress levels cause a weakening reflex in a muscle, thus making it vulnerable and more easily accessed. This, in turn, opens up other areas to be observed and examined. Patients with a large amount of physical strength cannot resist the brain's signal telling them that significant pain is found in a specific part of the body.

The process of Applied Kinesiology is the quickest and most efficient way of determining the cause, or underlying factors, of a health problem whether mental, emotional or physical. These issues disturb the harmony of the triangle of health by throwing off one or more parts of it. If someone is a non-believer in the processes of Applied Kinesiology, actual laboratory tests can be administered to provide hard evidence that the problem really does exist. Laboratory testing can provide additional information that may not be evident by applying Applied Kinesiology techniques. It can show that a more severe problem may be present requiring further medical attention or treatment. Alternative medicine isn't always the absolute answer to a problem as invasive procedures are foregone to

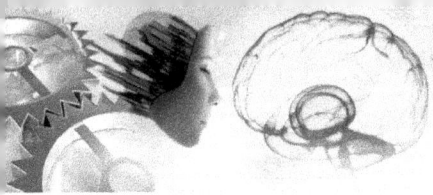

maintain a natural approach to healing. In some cases, non-holistic approaches must be taken in order to truly diagnose and treat a patient in the most appropriate manner. Applied Kinesiology can't always determine a severe condition. In serious cases, the apparent symptoms revealed during examination and treatment can disguise more severe conditions.

Mental/Emotional Aspects of

The Triangle of Health

Each side of our the triangle of health substantially affects the other two sides. The triangle mentioned previously is a metaphorical triangle (Improving Emotional Health, 2012). A harmonious balance occurs when all aspects of the triangle are healthy and intact. In order for this harmonious balance to occur, our structural, chemical and mental/emotional aspects must all be in proper health and balance.

Structural imperfections can be corrected with stretching, posture, and various exercises. There are many techniques available, including Neuro Emotional Technique, which involve building and strengthening emotions and health ties. Proper diet, avoidance, supplements and detoxification balance out our chemical health and strength. When all of these aspects are properly aligned and healthy, our body functions similar to a "well-oiled" machine.

A common misconception is that healthcare professionals can cure our emotional distress. They may aid in providing relief or a cure, but they do not cure it. *We* cure our own emotional distress. It is important to remember that part of human nature is to experience an emotional reaction to certain events, which

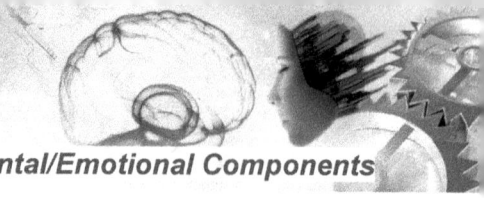

is perfectly acceptable. The way that we react to these instances is crucial. If we bottle up our emotions without properly handling them, we can suffer from a myriad of mental illnesses including Post-Traumatic Stress Disorder.

Returning to a healthy balance in a reasonable amount of time is what we need to focus on. When we store hurtful emotions and memories, our physiological balance is disrupted. We can prevent the manifestation of more serious or debilitating illnesses from occurring making healthy choices in all aspects of life affecting the triangle.

A recent study in neuroscience has proven that emotions are an interaction between chains of amino acids that form neuropeptides and receptors. What we do not realize is that emotions are organic processes that occur in the body naturally. Emotions can be both pleasant and unpleasant. We want to always keep the more positive emotions rather than allow detrimental emotions.

Imbalanced emotions can affect our physical health more than we expect them to. The wrong emotions can actually debilitate a person. Emotions do not stay within our minds; they are stored in many parts of our bodies. Acupuncturists in ancient times correlated emotions to specific organs in the body. Some of those correlations include, fear with the kidneys, anger with the liver and grief with the lungs. Predominantly, however, emotions are physiologically attached to our brains. Emotions are also automatically assumed to be stored in our spines, acupuncture circuits and autonomic nervous systems. Vast research has concluded that emotions travel to almost every cell in the body.

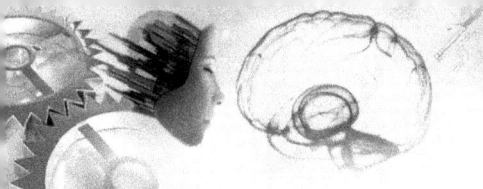

Emotions are very necessary and can be very good for us. Having emotions is healthy. It is important for us to feel differently in various situations. If we have no reaction at all, we are incapable of understanding a situation or knowing what it is to feel emotional stress or sadness. Although these are negative emotions, it is healthy to feel them. Feeling certain emotions can trigger memories from past events associated with a similar feeling. Not dwelling on previous emotions or events is a healthy process. A brief period of time to reflect on those events is sometimes necessary. Linking events can also be considered a reflex. This reflex is called a Pavlovian-type reflex. These reflexes are associations made within the mind to connect events or structure.

Dr. Scott Walker, a chiropractor from San Diego, California, developed N.E.T. or the Neuro Emotional Technique. He combined Traditional Chinese Medicine, chiropractic science and muscle testing to form the basis of his technique. The purpose for this testing was to determine a link or connection to the reflex pattern discussed in the Ivan Pavlov documentations. The development of this technique allowed Dr. Walker to access emotions that were associated with a reflex. N.E.T. is used to detect and reprogram negative memories. The process of reprogramming includes muscle reflexes/reactions, semantic reflexes, other muscle tests and body reflex points, all of which work to locate the origin of an event or an emotion's effect on the body. This process is used to normalize a neurological imbalance to improve physiological health. N.E.T. does not tell us what our plan of action has to be or should be; that part is up to us to figure out, N.E.T. strictly pertains to our physiological reaction to a past event.

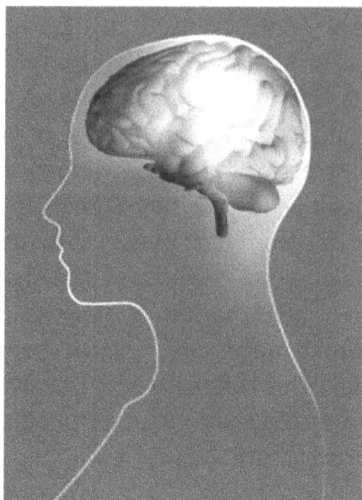

The Neuro Emotional Technique does not change the recollection of a previous event at all nor does it tell us what may have truly happened in the past. The Neuro Emotional Technique allows one to merely acknowledge a past event, whether it really happened or not. This technique triggers our own emotional reality because the events may have only occurred within our own minds and do not affect us in a physical manner. Our minds can contrive a situation from other events, making us think that a different situation actually occurred. For example, we may have had a deep emotional reaction to a vivid, fictional, dream.

Correcting our neuro-emotional complex is a safe process. . When the emotional side of the triangle is healthier, determining the needs of the structural and chemical sides becomes easier.

The layers of the structural, chemical and emotional sides of the triangle of health can be associated with the visual make up of

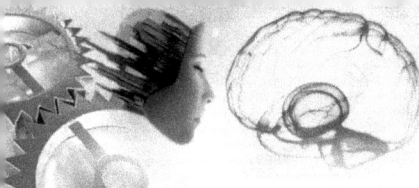

an artichoke. We peel the layers of an artichoke to get to the heart like we peel back the surface layers of a situation to get to the heart of the problem troubling us.

Some people that suffer from extreme mental or emotional distress are referred to a psychologist or other psychiatric professional for an evaluation or comprehensive treatment. The counseling, guidance and advice received from these professionals can help us release the negative emotional energy from our bodies to promote a healthy healing process. A professional may bring an underlying negative emotion to the forefront to tackle it directly. This therapy enables us to eliminate unhealthy, negative emotions and emotional energies. Some professional guidance can be quite beneficial in helping us on the path to a healthy mental and emotional state, and towards rebalancing the triangle of health.

The influence of Neuro Emotional Technique is limitless. There are no ceilings or barriers placed on the positive effects that the technique can have. N.E.T. maximizes our ability to remove conditioned reflexes and our optimal and overall mental and emotional health. Proper guidance and encouragement in utilizing the Neuro Emotional Technique helps put bad memories and events behind us in a healthy way.

Chiropractic Care and the Triangle of Health

Seeking Chiropractic care to aid in relieving physical, mental and structural health with non-prescription or non-invasive procedures aids in healing mental and emotional stresses. Sometimes spinal adjustments, acupuncture, holistic and natural nutritional supplements can be all that we need. An

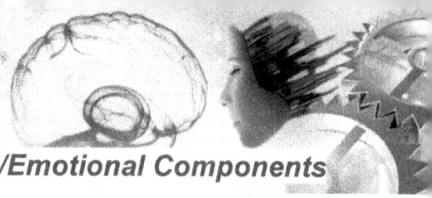

adjustment of our spine can relieve pressure-causing pain that may have been affecting our emotional health and can bring an immediate sense of happiness and stress relief (Improving Emotional Health, 2012). Stress on joints and muscles can cause anger and negative emotions that can be alleviated through the use of acupuncture. Aromatherapy coupled with acupuncture can be very soothing because a calm, relaxed environment of tranquil sounds and smells aids in the relaxation process.

Discuss in detail with a Chiropractor the exact problems that you are experiencing and how they may have started. Your muscle tension or body aches could have been caused by an emotionally traumatic event.

The structural side of the triangle of health is also important to maintain since it does affect the harmony of the emotional and chemical sides, and vice versa.

Combining Chiropractic Care, Applied Kinesiology, diet and exercise in proper balances gives us the results we seek (Applied Kinesiology Clinic, 2012). Feeling inadequate or incomplete can be more harmful to our bodies than we care to acknowledge.

Some may see a Chiropractic visit as unnecessary, but it is often amazing to see the apparent differences in such a person's body language and facial expressions after the visit.

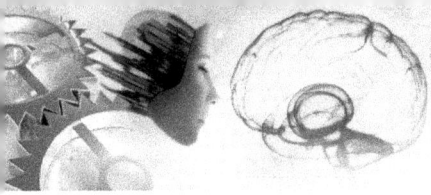

Chapter 2:

The Various Aspects of Stress and the Role of Chiropractic Care in Dealing with Them

Today, 'stress' has become a rather overused word. Commonly, it is used to denote a condition which creates physical and/or psychological pressure; however, it is not so easy to define. In fact, since the beginning of the usage of this term in biology, scientists have been searching unsuccessfully for the exact definition. Although the word is frequently used, the phenomenon itself and its mechanism are highly complicated. A historical as well as physiological perspective is necessary to truly understand the concept of stress.

Stress – a historical and biological perspective

A historical and biological perspective are both necessary in order to arrive at a meaningful definition of stress. This complex matter is further complicated by the fact that the concept of stress was being used in physics for a few centuries before the term was imported into biology.

In 1936, Hans Selye was conducting an experiment on laboratory animals. He observed that when the animals were exposed to negative physical stimuli like excessive noise, blaring light or thermal extremes, they developed certain common physical symptoms. These included stomach ulcers and enlargement of the adrenal glands. Thus, negative external stimuli caused physiological changes in the body.

Selye theorized that there are certain common physical conditions, such as heart attacks, strokes and kidney problems (among others), which may actually arise due to common external stimuli. These stimuli were defined as stress and covered many different aspects of it.

Selye defined stress as "the non-specific response of the body to any demand placed upon it". Scientists were soon looking for better alternatives but could not find any. The search became so frustrating that Selye finally described stress as something that, "in addition to being itself, was also the cause of itself, and the result of itself."

In order to understand the biological concept of stress, it is necessary to understand the idea of homeostasis. Broadly speaking, homeostasis means a state of balance. This is the ideal condition in which you should exist. Everything in your physique and your mind should be perfectly balanced and at rest.

The human responses are guided by two nervous systems: the sympathetic and the parasympathetic. The sympathetic nervous system takes your body to a level of high alert where you can trigger the classic fight or flight response. The parasympathetic nervous system helps in relaxation. A balance between the two will lead to homeostasis. However, when this balance is sometimes disturbed, one's body can feel "on edge" ready for fight or flight. This is the state of stress.

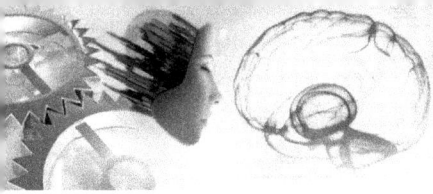

Though stress is a necessary biological trigger and does have a positive connotation, it is mostly used in the negative sense. It is a state of excessive physical, mental or emotional strain.

Perhaps the best modern definition for stress was given by Lazarus. It states that stress is "a condition or feeling experienced when a person perceives that demands exceed the personal and social resources the individual is able to mobilize."

The fact is that everybody knows what stress is, but it has been difficult to evolve a definition that is universally acceptable to the scientific community. It still remains largely a subjective concept and hence does not lend itself readily to quantitative studies.

Stress – good or bad?

The answer to the above query seems obvious. Stress is definitely bad. It gives rise to a number of medical conditions – both chronic and acute, which may even lead to death. However, the matter is not always that simple. Stress has both a positive and a negative side, and the former is actually necessary.

Stress is necessary for human beings to perform optimally. Stimuli which cause stress will cause the body to be more productive so that optimal results are achieved. For many, the stress of anticipating a big test, sporting event, performance, or other event drives students to excel. This good stress is known as eustress.

It is possible to have either acute eustress or chronic eustress. Chronic eustress is a continued feeling of happiness and satisfaction. This is difficult to achieve and yet should be the

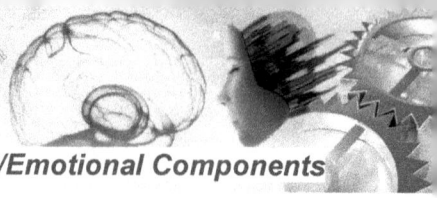

goal of every life. During this state, the chemical compounds in your body are at optimal levels and they allow you to function in the best possible way. Acute eustress is felt when there is a sudden spurt of intense happiness or satisfaction within a very short time. So, if you receive excellent news suddenly, you will experience acute eustress.

When your body is subjected to these good stresses, 'feel good' hormones like dopamine and oxytocin flood your bloodstream.

However, the negative connotation of stress is much better known. This category is called distress and it too can be acute or chronic.

Acute distress is intense, rapid and short lived. It floods the physical system with emergency response hormones like adrenaline and cortisol. These cause your levels of alertness, endurance and energy to increase. This system is necessary to help deal with various emergencies that you may face in the course of your life.

The worst type of stress is chronic distress; a long, enduring state of distress where the body always contains an excess of emergency response hormones. On the other hand, the 'feel good' hormones are suppressed. The entire endocrine system is overused. Chronic distress is the most important cause of the various physiological conditions commonly associated with stress.

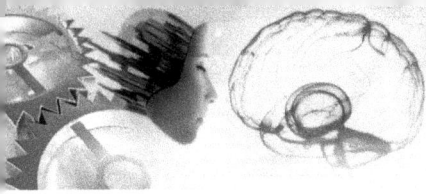

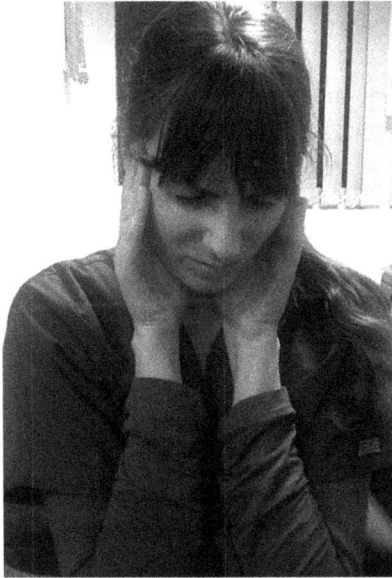

A woman suffering from a tension headache

There are two other categories of stress known as hyperstress and hypostress. Both are negative in nature. Hyperstress refers to an extreme condition which pushes the human body to its limit. Such a condition may arise during extreme pain like labor. On the other hand, hypostress refers to an opposite situation. It is a situation of inactivity and boredom which can induce fatigue and eventually lead to depression.

The types of stress according to origin

Stress in the human body can arise from many different factors. These can broadly be grouped into four types. There are structural stress, chemical stress, thermal stress and finally emotional stress. The mechanism is described below:

Structural stress

The stresses that arise in the human body due to structural factors are categorized as structural stress.

The human body may be so aligned that the neuro-musculo-skeletal structure is not optimum. This can trigger stress.

Such structural problems may be caused by many different factors. Some people suffer from congenital problems which interfere with the structure of the body. For example, people who suffer from deformities of the skull caused by faulty suturing are victims of structural stress.

Certain diseases or injuries can also give rise to structural stress. Any strains, sprains, nerve injuries or fractures can cause structural stress.

Conditions like herniated discs, arthritis and osteophytes seriously interfere with the structure of the human body and give rise to stress.

Structural stress can arise not only from the skeletal system but also from the muscles and nerves of the body. Weak muscles, pinched or stretched nerves and postural imbalances can all lead to structural stress.

The most common symptom is pain, though it may not be acute or instant. This may be accompanied by weakness, phobia and loss of confidence.

Chemical stress

Any stress that is introduced in the body by chemical means can be regarded as chemical stress.

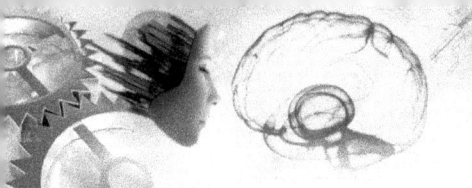

Chemicals enter the human body through food, drink and anything else that you may consume. Consumption of items which contain undesirable chemicals will surely lead to chemical stress. No wonder it is said that you are what you eat.

One significant method by which undesirable chemicals are often introduced in the body is through prescription drugs. While they may be effective immediately, they often release a number of undesirable elements within the chemical structure of the human body. In most cases, the human body is able to neutralize these elements. However, as long as the chemicals stay within the body, they create chemical stress. The greatest strain of chemical stress is put on the kidneys because their primary function is to clean the body of undesirable and potentially toxic chemicals.

Alcohol, tobacco, and foods rich in sugar, caffeine, and cholesterol can introduce chemical stress into the body. Strangely enough, people seem to prefer eating fast food or candy when under stress aggravating the situation.

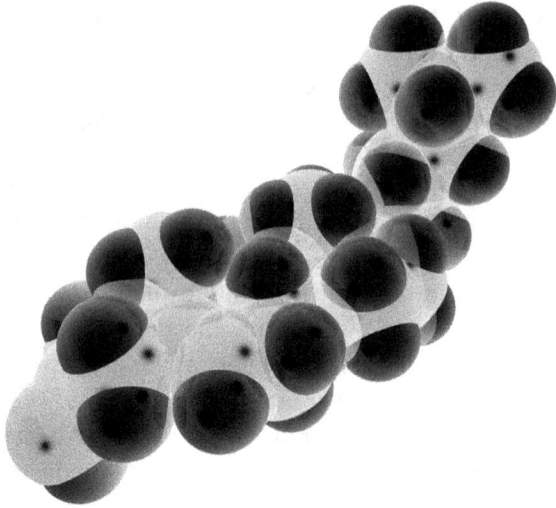

Cholesterol, such as the molecule shown above, can contribute to chemical stress on the body

Other factors can also contribute to chemical stress. Chemicals are released in the body by the endocrine system via hormones. These are biochemical substances that are targeted towards particular cells or organs causing specific changes. Hormones are secreted by glands. The adrenal gland most directly controls the release of hormones that deal with emergency situations in the body triggering the fight or flight response. Hormones like epinephrine, norepinephrine and adrenaline are released to help trigger an emergency response. Neural pathways join in the effort. All these changes occur within seconds, and the person is ready to fight for his or her life.

If a person is under stress, these hormone levels never return to normal. The continuous presence of stress factors heightens the chemical imbalance in the body, chemical stress becomes acute and the body is unable to return to its state of balance.

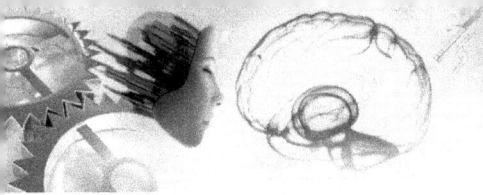

Thermal stress

The total heat that a person has to endure is called heat stress or thermal stress.

This heat comes from three different sources. These are the environment, work a person performs and, clothing a person wears.

The most comfortable range of heat tolerance of the human body is between 68°F to 81°F (20°C to 27°C) and for relative humidity this range is between 35% and 60%.

When the temperature of the external environment increases, more blood is pumped to the skin in order to stimulate the production of more sweat to regulate body temperature.

The human body gains heat by the following processes:

The human body gains metabolic heat through the process of food digestion.

It gains heat from radiation of surrounding hot objects like furnace pipes.

It gains heat from the atmosphere through the process of convection,

Some heat exchange also occurs through conduction and breathing.

As temperature increases, the body has to work harder to regulate its own temperature. Blood flow increases and its capacity for work declines with increased sweating. Thermal stress sets in.

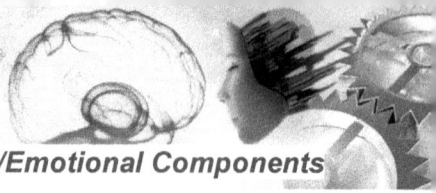

This thermal stress can lead to many different medical conditions ranging from heat rash, heat edema, and heat exhaustion to heat stroke and hyperpyrexia.

Long term thermal stress can lead to sleep disturbances, chronic heat exhaustion and susceptibility to injuries. It is also thought that long term heat exposure leads to a decrease in sperm count. Constant exposure to infrared rays is one of the leading causes of cataract.

Emotional stress

This is arguably the single most dominant type of stress affecting human beings today.

There are no visible or distinct symptoms of emotional stress. As a result, it becomes difficult to understand or identify who is suffering from emotional stress and exactly how much harm it is doing. In certain cases, however, emotional stress manifests itself in the form of tension headaches or even ulcers.

The modern lifestyle is a major cause of emotional stress. The economic situation of the world coupled with the pressures of a consumerist society creates lots of emotional stress.

The workplace has become another common cause of stress. With unemployment and layoffs on the rise, uncertainty and insecurity has increased. This creates a lot of workplace-related stress.

The security of personal relationships is no longer absolute. Breakdown in the structure of the family, abuse, drugs and alcohol are other major causes of emotional stress.

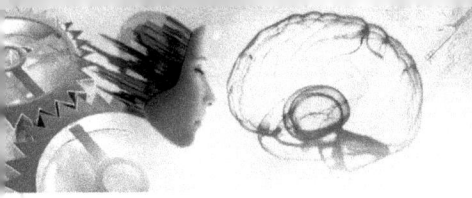

Likewise, peer pressure, competition and parental expectations have created a marked rise in emotional stress among today's adolescents.

Every person has his own emotional triggers which may lead to stress. Scientists have observed that the same event may create stress in one person and not in another. This phenomenon has been beautifully illustrated with an analogy. Consider a roller coaster ride. Those who ride in front scream and laugh and hop on the next ride as soon as this one ends. The riders at the back are clutching the security rail with white knuckles and tightly shut eyes, vowing never to get on another ride in their lives. So the two groups have two different perceptions of the same event. The situation was stimulating to the former group while it creating both physical and emotional stress in the latter.

In 1968, Mason carried out an experiment on people performing stressful activities by measuring the level of stress hormones in their blood before and after exposure to stressful activity. From his study he concluded that when a person faces a novel or unpredictable situation over which he has no perceivable control, emotional stress occurs and stress hormones are released. Threat to the ego is another type of situation that has the same result.

Persistence of emotional stress can lead to several complications. There is a definite increase in moodiness and forgetfulness and natural abilities are hampered. It can eventually lead to sleep disorders and insomnia as well as eating disorders. Chronic emotional stress has been known to impair the reproductive abilities in both men and women.

Chronic emotional stress has an impact on the endocrine system, neurotransmitters, metabolic rate and enzymes. It may lead to a number of diseases ranging from ulcers to heart disease.

The interrelationship between the four types of stress

The four types of stress described above are distinct and separate as far as causative factors are concerned. However, there is a close interrelationship among the four of them. This arises from the fact that regardless of the cause of the stress, the human body has certain set responses to it. This implies that the body reacts in a particular way as soon as it is subjected to stress. The intensity of this reaction is different in the case of acute and chronic stress. However, whether it arises from structural, chemical, thermal or emotional causes, the reaction is very similar, though somewhat different.

The interrelationship can be described in the following way:

The stress response in the human body is controlled by the limbic brain. This is the mid level portion of the brain and has been described as the emotional control center.

When the brain perceives a situation as stressful, the limbic brain sends signals to activate the hypothalamus – pituitary – adrenal axis. The hypothalamus activates the autonomous nervous system, secretes vasopressin and also stimulates the thyroid gland. However, its main function is to secrete hormones that release corticotrophin. This in turn stimulates the pituitary gland (located in the limbic brain) to secrete adrenocorticotropin hormone (ACTH). This hormone travels via blood vessels to stimulate the adrenal glands which are located over the kidneys. The adrenal glands finally release stress

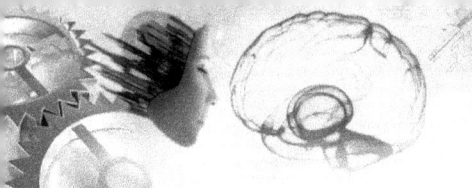

hormones into the blood. Cortisols, epinephrine and norepinephrine are the main stress hormones.

Whether the stress is structural, chemical, thermal or emotional, this hormonal response is common to all.

The best way to perceive the interrelation between the different types of stress can be seen in the physical and psychological effects of stress. Structural stress developed in the region of the cervical vertebra will trigger pain and numbness. The common prescriptions for this are painkillers and non-steroidal anti-inflammatory drugs (NSAIDs) such as ibuprofen or aspirin. They often release strong chemicals in the body adding chemical stress to your structural stress. Moreover, emotional stress is always present, even though the primary cause of stress may be different. So, persons under thermal stress easily lose their temper.

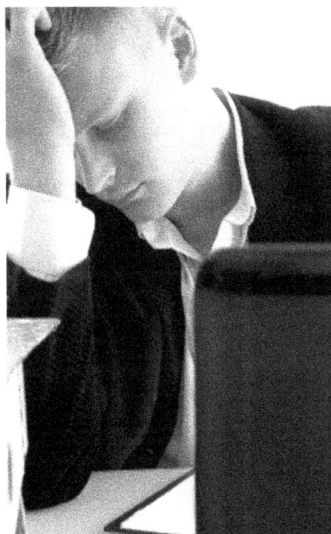

The fact remains that there is still a lot left to know and understand about the phenomenon of stress, its causes and its measurements. As more studies are undertaken, the exact mechanism of mutual influence and interaction between different types of stress will become more evident.

The effects of stress

The impact of stress is not restricted to an increased heartbeat and profuse sweating for the first few minutes. Though extensive scientific evidence is still to be collected, stress is thought to have serious implications for quite a few physical and psychological maladies.

- Stress is directly responsible for increase in unhealthy practices such as the ingestion of tobacco, alcohol and drugs, including prescription medicines.
- Stress reactions cause blood pressure to increase as the heartbeat increases. The blood thickens in preparation for possible injury. Inflammatory markers are released in the bloodstream. All these significantly increase the risk of stroke and heart disease.
- Stress cardiomyopathy is a commonly observed phenomenon, especially in men. The symptoms imitate a heart attack as does the EKG, but no blockage or coronary malfunction is ever detected.
- Chronic stress compromises the immune system of the body.
- Certain digestive disorders like peptic ulcers, irritable bowel syndrome and inflammatory bowel disease are aggravated considerably by stress.

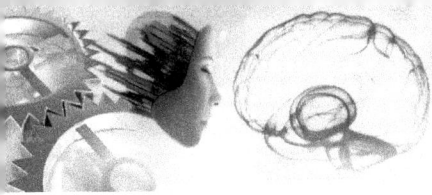

- Stress probably has a strong link with various eating disorders and obesity, though conclusive studies are yet to be done.
- Diabetes and insomnia are common side effects of stress.
- The earliest signal of stress is pain. Tension headaches are the most common indication. Muscular and neural pain is also common, especially in structural stress.
- Reproductive functions like sperm count, premenstrual syndrome, and menopause have a definite link to stress.
- The effects of stress are seen in numerous skin diseases, hair loss, memory loss and even in the degeneration of the gums and teeth.

Recent researches have established strong links between stress and cancer. In a study, Professor Tian Xu of Yale University concluded that stress opens up pathways in the cancer causing mutations that occur in different cells to speed up the disease. Emotional or physical stress first begins to affect sleep, which in turn restricts the production of melatonin in the body. This enzyme plays a key role in supressing cancer. Stress also suppresses the immune system, followed by a release of adrenal hormones in the body. The latter occur because of excess production of the stress hormone. The glucose levels rise drastically within the cells; pathogens make these cells their host and their intervention helps in creating cancerous cells. An increased level of stress hormones leads to the increase of this cancerous mass.

Stress and modern medicine

Though it is difficult to define and isolate stress, the above discussion clearly shows that stress plays an important role in the health of modern human beings. It has been identified as the leading proxy killer of America, increasing the chances of stroke and heart disease. Not only that, but $200 to $300 billion is lost every year through stress related causes.

However, if we study the role that modern medicine plays in the management of stress, it must be said that this insidious illness has not received the attention that it deserves. Till recent times, stress was not considered a significant entity. Even today, there is no universally acknowledged definition of this problem.

Modern medicine has, however, developed certain methods for measuring stress. These are as follows:

Several psychological questionnaires have been developed to understand and measure stress levels.

Blood pressure is taken as another measure of stress.

A study conducted by Li and Gleeson (2004) and Walsh (1999) indicates that measurement of the alpha-amylase enzyme in the saliva can be used as a measurement of stress because this enzyme is produced in greater quantities when the sympathetic nervous system becomes active.

Measurement of level of cortisols in the saliva and blood is another measure of levels of stress.

You might notice that that whatever efforts have been made in this direction are all very recent. In fact, traditional medicine historically paid little attention to stress. Even today, the means of measurement clearly show that the concern remains with chemical stress. However, it is emotional stress which is playing a more prominent role in affecting human health. The medical community acknowledges the impact of emotional stress on the human body as well as on its sub-systems, such as blood

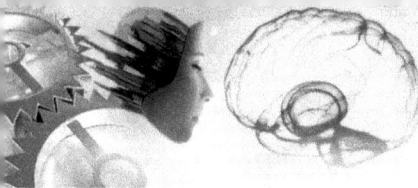

circulation, the nervous system, sleep and the reproductive system. Still, there have been few serious efforts to study them.

In the changing world scenario of today, emotional stress has become a highly worrying factor. In fact, the University of London conducted a study over 20 years. It concluded that stress, if left unmanaged, contributes more to heart disease and cancer than tobacco or foods high in cholesterol. Yet, modern medical science has failed to designate appropriate importance to stress and the prescription remains comparable to what it was two to three decades ago.

Chiropractic care for stress

In the absence of any strong positive action by traditional medicine, people are turning more and more to alternative medicine for stress relief. Yoga and acupuncture are now established alternative remedies for stress.

Chiropractic care can greatly help in the reduction and management of stress. The following points help explain the connection between chiropractic care and stress:

Chiropractic cannot remove the stressors. This means that chiropractic care will not be able to remove those elements in your environment that are the actual cause of your emotional stress. However, if it is a question of structural or chemical stress, chiropractic care can definitely eliminate that.

The theory of chiropractic care for stress management is simple. Whether you are feeling stress due to structural, chemical or thermal reasons, you will become aware of the stress through pain. Pain is the earliest signal that your body sends you to indicate something is wrong. This pain is conveyed to you via the nerves. Chiropractic care recommends intercepting this pain in the nerve and then gradually working backwards so that the physical symptoms of stress are ultimately eliminated.

The spinal cord is the central receiving station of all the information conveyed by the nerves. So, all stress is finally relayed to the spinal cord and the vertebra. This will definitely hamper the normal orientation of the vertebra. This situation is known as spinal subluxation.

Chiropractors use the principles of movement and reflexes to deal with stress. Movement implies the full range of musculoskeletal movement that a particular part of the body can perform. When performed correctly, the nervous system will work in an efficient manner and will be able to largely neutralize the stress factor.

The phenomenon of reflex often causes stress in one part of the body to be conveyed to another part of the body in a different form. Tension headaches are the best examples. Cervical vertebrae being out of alignment creates structural stress which is converted into tension headaches. Chiropractic principles utilize this property of the human body. Instead of prescribing painkillers for the headache that only add to the chemical stress in the body, chiropractors use the principle of reflex. The structural stress is corrected by different processes and the tension headache disappears by itself. Brain balancing is one chiropractic technique which has been seen to be especially helpful in stress management. It emphasizes a set of exercises called cross crawls and pressure on reflex points situated below the collarbones.

Chiropractors suggest a number of relaxation techniques to tackle the problem of emotional stress. All this stress actually

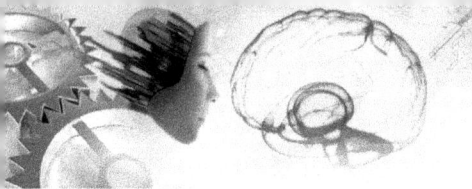

manifests itself in your nerves, which ultimately find their way to the spine. Breaking down the spine into sections and adjusting them by touch so that they are back in alignment will significantly reduce stress.

More and more people report that chiropractic treatment has helped them to deal with stress-induced problems like sleep deprivation, tension headaches, irritability and forgetfulness.

Much more research has to be done in order to fully understand the phenomenon of stress, its causes, effects, and ways to control it. In the meantime, chiropractic care has utilized the body's ability to heal itself to reverse the effects of stress to a very large extent.

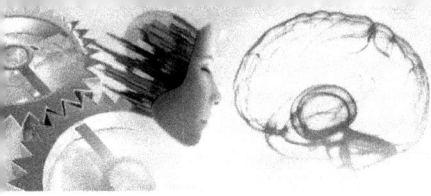

Chapter 3:

Emotions and Emotional State

What is Emotion?

Emotion can be summed up in three terms; observable behavior, expressed feelings and changes in the body's state. Emotion is hard to study due to it being so complex and diverse. Emotion is very personal and can be difficult to define or identify at times. Simple emotions can often appear to be more complicated than they really are.

In one instance, emotion is defined as a feeling that is private and subjective. Sometimes, obvious indicators are not present when someone is experiencing emotional distress (Infinite Minds, 2012). Their behavior may appear normal to their individual personality. Also, there are times someone tries to imitate or "blend" with another so well that emotional distress is not recognized.

Emotion is a state of psychological arousal, or, in more scientific terms, a display of somatic or autonomic response. This suggests that specific emotional states can be defined by specific groups of bodily responses affecting mostly the heart and stomach.

Emotions are often characterized as defending or attacking in response to a threat. This element of emotion ties into Darwin's point of view of the functional roles of emotion. Darwin's study indicates that emotions have an important role in survival because they generate action in dangerous situations.

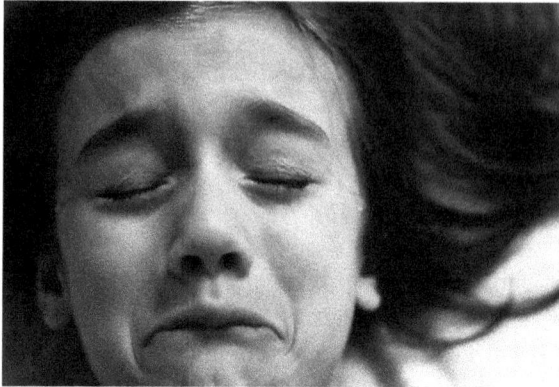

Categories

Psychologists have attempted to break emotions up into categories. Wilhelm Wundt, a 19th Century Psychologist, suggested that emotions are grouped in three basic dimensions with pairs of opposite views. Examples of this would be pleasantness/unpleasantness, tension/release and excitement/relaxation. With more exploration and over time, these pairings and other discoveries became more complex. Plutchik, another Psychologist, asserted that there are actually eight basic emotions grouped into four pairs. Those pairs are joy/sadness, acceptance/disgust, anger/fear and surprise/anticipation. When people are asked how they feel, one of the above options is a common answer.

Emotion can also be defined as a spontaneous reaction to a given circumstance. These responses and feelings vary from person to person. They are perception-based and are subjective to individual experiences. Therapeutic help is sought when

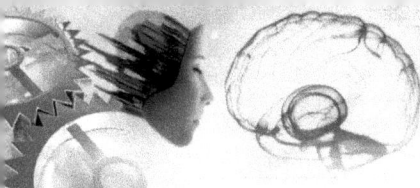

people are unable to handle the flow of their emotions, or the intense feelings they bring on. A person may seek out the help of a professional to aid them in understanding their feelings and where they come from.

There are primary and secondary emotions. The primary emotions are the first ones that we feel in response to an action or circumstance. This is our initial response. Secondary emotions then take over and mask our initial feelings. Secondary emotions make it harder to distinguish problems and properly work through them.

Emotional and Mental states are as different as they are similar. There is a distinct difference between them, although they are often confused. Emotions are feelings such as happy, sad, depressed, anxious and so on. A mental state of health determines a chemical imbalance within our brains that generally cause psychiatric disorders such as bipolar disorder and schizophrenia. Depression is one mental disorder that can be treated like an emotional disorder. It can cause us to malfunction in our daily lives just as other mental disorders do, but it is often treatable with the use of NET. Other mental disorders often require medication and extensive psychotherapy.

Theories of Emotion

Theories of emotion are mostly based on physiology, thought and the actual emotion itself. Basic questions are asked to help distinguish or establish the reasoning for the emotion to be felt.

These basic questions are:

• In what order do these occur?

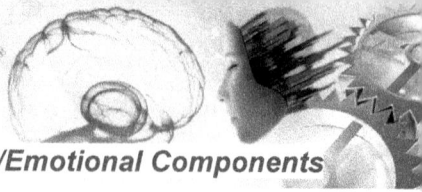

• Do we think a certain way because of the emotions that we feel or vice versa?

• Do we feel emotions because of how we perceive the body's actions?

• Do we have a physical reaction because of the emotions we feel?

Physiological, neurological and cognitive categories are singled out as theories of motivation when sorting out emotions. The Physiological theories suggest that responses within our bodies are responsible for our emotions. Neurological theories suggest that brain activity leads to certain emotional responses. Cognitive theories place thoughts and mental activity at the forefront of the formation of emotions.

There are three main theories of emotion to explain emotion and emotional reactions. Those theories are the opinions of the teams of James and Lange, Cannon and Bard and Schachter and Singer. The theory of James and Lange is by far the best known theory of emotion. It discusses the fact that when you are scared, your body shows this emotion by trembling. The Cannon-Bard Theory suggests that we are capable of experiencing more than one reaction to an emotion at once. We experience sweating, muscle tension and trembling at the same time in response to an event. The final theory examined is the Schachter-Singer theory. This theory discusses the idea that physiological arousal occurs first. We must then identify the arousal and determine the emotion behind it.

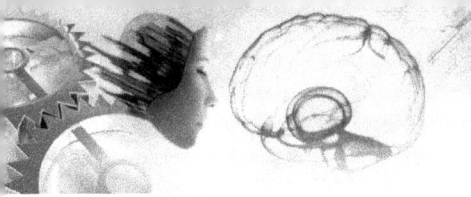

Emotions and Your Diet

It may not seem like a reasonable correlation, but our diets are often controlled by the emotions that we feel. Our food choices, or cravings, can stem from the way that we feel. For instance, if we are feeling sad we are likely to choose a food option that is heavy, comforting and filling such as pasta or starch. Some will associate sadness with craving something soothing such as chocolate or peanut butter. Eating is often associated with feelings of punishment, pleasure, pain or sadness. We rarely reward ourselves with food when we are happy. The emotion of fear of gaining weight steers us away from eating foods that may be fattening.

Emotions and dietary choices go hand in hand. They can determine each other quite easily.

We sometimes eat because we are sad or are sad because we ate something that, perhaps, we shouldn't have. Foods that interact negatively with blood sugar levels can induce the

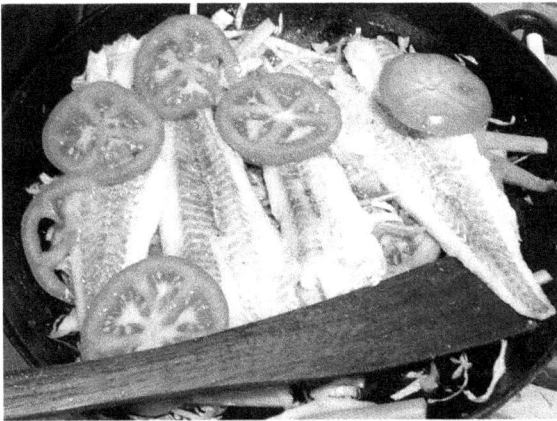

emotion of irritability or depression. Oddly enough, food allergies can provoke emotional outbursts.

Increased sugar levels causing depression or irritability can be reversed by increasing water intake or going for a brisk walk. Sugar boosts our metabolism allowing us extra energy for exercise. Burning the sugar off with exercise can be spiritually and emotionally relaxing. Children are more susceptible to irritability and emotional outbursts due to increased sugar levels and the increased intake of impurities often found in processed or manufactured foods. Reducing or completely removing these items from your family's diet will promote the overall emotional health and stability of the family. Happy children generally grow into happy adults.

When we consume pure and high quality food items, we are able to maintain a healthy emotional balance. Sub-standard food items can disrupt our systems, causing an emotional imbalance. Foods that are high in fat place massive demands upon the digestive system, and divert blood away from the brain. This interferes with our emotions to some degree. Our brains feeling sluggish can bring forth a feeling of depression.

Dramatic emotional disturbances are displayed when a poorly balanced diet is consumed. This includes a lot of foods that are high in sugar, fat, salt and carbohydrates. Fluctuations in emotions will then be displayed more frequently. Philosophers have even categorized what certain foods can do to specific emotional states.

Foods affect our mental and emotional states in two ways. The first is that they either replenish or deplete vital nutrients that our mental and emotional health depends on. The second is

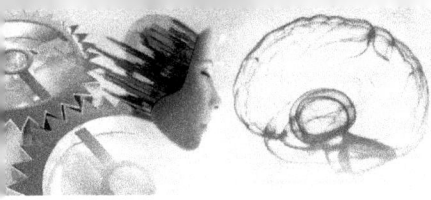

that toxic byproducts are produced by the food that can poison the brain, leading to emotional problems.

Emotion and Your Health

Staying healthy requires healthy emotions as well as a healthy body. Many people have difficulty maintaining healthy emotions. It is not often a physiological disorder but a misinterpretation of who we really are. Negative emotions are toxic to our bodies because they are destructive to our mental and physical wellbeing. It has been noted and proven that someone suffering from emotional distress can have frequent backaches and headaches, often leading to migraines.

Toxic emotions can often be stored and not released. They can deter us from maintaining proper health. Unhappiness can lead to long-term health problems that may have an irreversible effect. Continuous or prolonged exposure to unhealthy situations or people can result in us being caught in a web of toxic emotions (our emotional health intelligence emotion, 2012). To alleviate this problem, we need to backtrack a little bit. We need to figure out where the emotions first began, what triggered them, and what the environmental situation was. Identifying this factor can set a person on the path to recuperation and healing. Decipher, within yourself, how you could have reacted differently to that situation. Satisfy your mind with your findings and release the negative emotions from your thoughts. This will help the negative toxins that they have produced to subside, and eventually, will deplete them completely. The most common term for this experience is called trapped emotions. Trapped emotions can incapacitate us. They can take over our very existence, making it impossible for us to function in a productive manner.

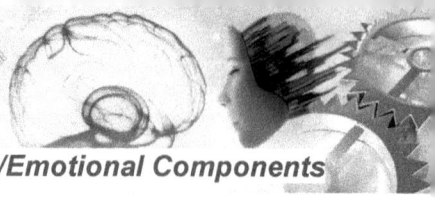

Releasing your body of negative toxins or negative emotions must be done via a slow process. Negative emotions cause stress, which needs to be alleviated and reduced gradually in order to make us less susceptible to other ailments. We should always try to go to bed at night with a clear mind that is at ease. A troubled mind can cause violent dream sequences, interrupted sleep patterns and angry feelings upon waking. If you feel like you did not get any rest and wake up still tired from the day before, a look at your emotional health is in order. It may be a helpless feeling to have these emotions in the back of your mind all of the time, but there is something you can do about it. It requires primarily, the desire to improve your mental, emotional and physical health, along with definite, though small steps in the right directions. Help from a therapist may be needed to help guide you in initiating healthy thought processes and healthy reactions to situations. It will also help to teach you what triggers negative emotions, and how to counteract them into becoming healthy, positive emotions.

Some substances are also known to be able to alter our emotional state. Caffeine, alcohol and illicit drugs can have significant effects on our mental state. Caffeine is a stimulant that can, when consumed in large amounts, trigger a panic attack or general anxiety-like feeling. Alcohol and illicit drugs reduce our capacity to react in a realistic manner to events. These substances can induce violent or angry tendencies, bringing on stress and sadness.

Many of us may not realize it, but some of the foods that we eat can distort how we perceive things. Yes, foods can contribute to the way we feel. These distortions mostly come from food additives and foods that are not pure. Vitamin and nutrient deficiencies can also play a part in emotional distress. Our brains can be deprived of components essential to the release

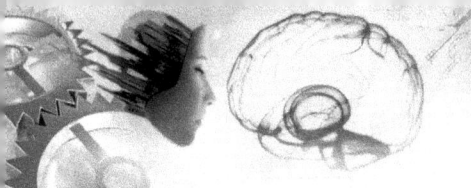

of happy emotions. Magnesium, calcium, potassium and Vitamin B complex are necessary elements for maintaining brain and emotional health. Increased or over-consumption of sugar is detrimental to the maintenance of the health of the brain.

Instabilities and imbalances in our emotional and/or mental states can cause a variety of other health problems that can be structural, chemical or emotional. It is a common misconception that the three are not linked when, in fact, they are essential in diagnosing a specific problem. Depression can be linked to chronic pain or to a chronic illness. In return, this chronic pain can cause hormonal imbalances in our brains. When this happens, signals can be crossed making us feel sad or depressed. It can also lead us to have other negative emotional disturbances. According to the Triangle of Health, when either one's structural, chemical or emotional sides are out of line it throws off the pattern of health in one's entire body.

Reversing the effects of negative emotional toxins in the brain is not an immediate process (Theories about emotion, 2012). You may want to build a support system of people that believe in you for that extra push to succeed. Encouragement often does the most good when it comes from an outside source. When others see how hard you are working to improve your moods and mental health, the environment around all of you becomes that much more peaceful and enjoyable. It takes time, patience, determination and the will to do so. The end result will find you experiencing more joy, and the ability to enjoy life to its fullest potential.

Statistics for Americans Regarding Emotional Instability

Americans are known for suffering from more emotional and mental distress than any other population around the world. Much of their emotional instability stems from not dealing with a traumatic or tragic event in their past. It can also come from ignoring illnesses, injuries or body pain. About one in five children in the United States between the ages of three and twelve suffer from emotional disturbances. An astonishing 70% of these children will not receive medical attention for these disturbances.

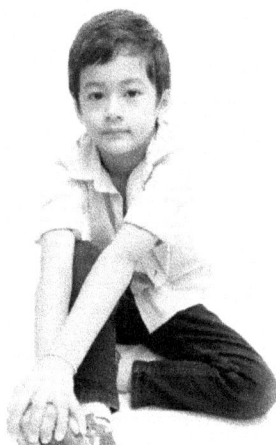

It is also estimated that 57.7% of American adults suffer from an emotional or mental disorder. Specifically, 6.7% of American adults suffer from Depression. Suicide is the 11th leading cause of death in the United States and thousands of lives are claimed by suicide stemming from emotional or mental distress every year.

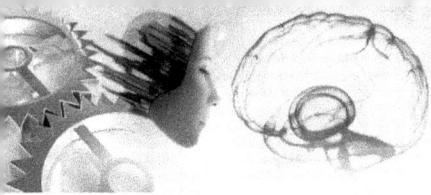

It is said that 90% of suicide victims have a treatable and undiagnosed emotional or mental disorder.

Treatments for Emotional Health and Stability

There are different treatment options to ensure emotional health and stability. One's course of action will vary depending on the severity of their issues. It is suggested that a journal be started to note changes in one's emotional state. These entries should include what the circumstances were, what emotion you feel, when it starts and any other circumstances that played a role in a mood change. If you began to feel irritable after eating a lot of sugar, it should be noted. A detailed mood diary can help us to establish how negative emotions are triggered and if there is a pattern to the way we feel at times.

Alternative and mainstream treatment options are available to treat emotional health and stability (DeAngelis, T, 2012). It is up to you and your doctor as to what avenue to explore first. It may take more than one option to help de-escalate your issues Treatments for maintaining sound emotional health include acupuncture, massage therapy, chiropractic care and Applied Kinesiology. Alternative medicine is ultimately the best way to treat emotional difficulties. These treatments teach you techniques to solve a problem without the use of harmful prescription drugs. Alternative medicine includes the use of natural supplements, dietary changes, muscle therapy, acupuncture and basic non-evasive chiropractic care is therefore a more healthy path to realign the emotional side of the Triangle of Health.

Neuro Emotional Technique

Neuro Emotional Technique or NET is described as a combination of techniques derived from traditional Chinese medicine, Applied Kinesiology and chiropractic care. It focuses on deficiencies in our nutrition, negative emotional blocks, toxins in the body and structural imbalances in our skeletomuscular systems. NET is a holistic approach to curing emotional and mental health problems. NET helps to release and resolve issues in our bodies known as negative emotional complexes, or NEC (Emotion in Psychology, 2012). This technique was developed in the 1980's by a chiropractor, Scott Walker. Walker performed several studies to conclude that NET helped to reduce the stress levels in a majority of the patients studied, thus making them happier overall.

Included in these studies were the applications of Applied Kinesiology and dietary changes. NET has been proven to reduce infertility stress, reduce or alleviate symptoms of Separation Anxiety Disorder and help patients with chronic pain. An astounding 88% of patients that used neuro emotional technique noticed a drastic amount of improvement.

There is a direct correlation between mental instability, emotional instability and chronic pain. In many cases, they tie together and have at their root one existing problem within the body. A person suffering from chronic neck pain, for example, can have this pain due to emotional and/or mental distress caused from a tragic or traumatic event in their life that remains unresolved. Another example would be a person feeling depressed by reason of having experienced years of chronic pain.

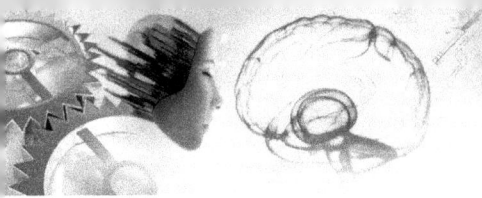

Lifestyle Changes

A change in your lifestyle may be just what the doctor ordered in terms of repairing your emotional health. Eating a balanced diet, exercising and getting into a strict sleep routine will aid your overall emotional health. Do your best to avoid high stress situations. Increase natural or raw food intake as much as possible. Decrease your intake of unhealthy items such as alcohol and excessive sugar. These small changes in your lifestyle can make a world of difference to your emotional health and stability. A move to a more tranquil environment may be in order.

We may not take into consideration the fact that our careers could be causing some of our emotional distress. Some jobs are very high maintenance, technically difficult or emotionally demanding. Our lifestyle outside of our career must be relaxed and enjoyable. If it is found that your career is causing your mental distress, it may be time to consider a brief hiatus from the position just to get your body back in proper alignment. Your job performance may be poor due to the dissatisfaction you experience with your current position. Seek out other opportunities or explore a hidden passion. Many people in technically demanding fields find that they enjoy painting, sculpting or even cooking. Try your hand at something new. There may be a new found joy that makes your career seem a little easier to cope with.

Drug Treatments

Mood swings or emotional distress can stem from an underlying health problem. A doctor can prescribe medications to aid in correcting the underlying problem in hopes of correcting both

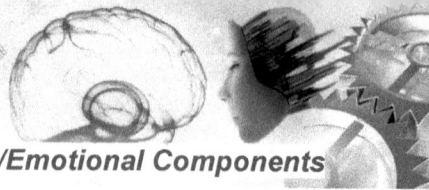

problems with one treatment option. Anti-depressants are the most common medications prescribed for treating mood swings. However, it is known that these can have adverse side effects. If you experience severe adverse side effects from a prescribed medication, discuss alternative medicine options with your prescribing doctor. In some cases, adding an nutritional supplement to a medication regimen can help to reverse or calm some of the adverse side effects.

Women entering menopause can often suffer from severe mood swings. This can alter one's emotional state, causing instability. Adding a hormone replacement therapy may be the best option. Hormone imbalances can definitely alter one's personality and emotional state. Hormone replacement therapy can be completely safe when it is properly administered. Discuss the risks of these treatments and their potential for causing certain types of cancer with your Physician first.

Before resorting to man-made drug treatments for emotional health and stability issues, consider herbal or natural options. Some natural supplements can be more beneficial to one's emotional health and stability without the adverse side effects of many prescription medications. These side effects can include decreased sexual desire, weight gain, headaches and even the risk of suicidal tendencies.

Psychological Treatments

Psychotherapy treatment sessions can be greatly beneficial in tackling emotional health problems. Discussing our problems and having aid in getting through them is a great release. The relief of stress that sometimes comes from just talking about a troublesome problem can sometimes be almost immediate. One Psychological aspect that we don't often consider is

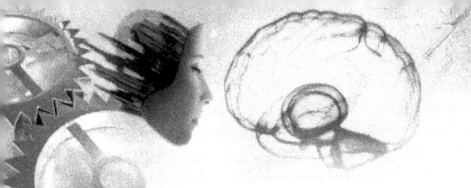

Cognitive Behavioral Therapy. This teaches us that we control our emotions. How we react to situations is up to us on a subconscious level. If we have control over our mental health, our emotional health will also benefit. With therapy, you'll be taught how to take a negative situation and end it with a positive result through the use of positive reinforcement and situation analysis exercises. These take some time to perfect, but with practice, a less stressful you is on the horizon.

Natural, Herbal and Homeopathic Remedies

The overall health of our nervous system, which ties into our emotional health and stability, can be boosted with the addition of natural, herbal and homeopathic remedies. Certain salts, including Natrium sulphate, Kalium sulphate and Natrium phosphate are biochemic salts that support our nervous systems (Heartburn Home Remedies, 2012). They lift our moods and reduce our anxiety levels. Salts such as those previously mentioned, are perfectly safe for children, pregnant women and nursing mothers to take. Herbal ingredients, including St. John's Wort and Passiflora, are proven to significantly reduce depression and anxiety, and to significantly uplift moods. Folic Acid and Omega-3 Fatty Acids are also beneficial in the healing and maintaining of healthy emotions.

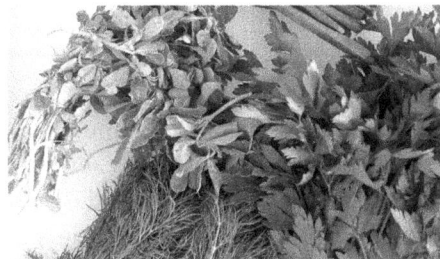

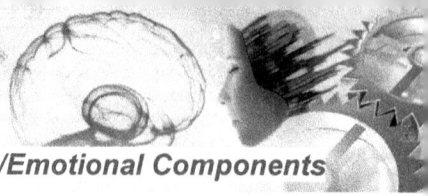

Seeking the help of an alternative medicine healthcare professional for a properly balanced diet can be beneficial. Learning what foods to eat and what foods to avoid can make all of the difference in the world.

Eating better makes you feel better, which brings your body's natural endorphins to life. When our endorphins come to life, we experience happy emotions.

Aromatherapy is a great homeopathic way to soothe our minds and reduce levels of stress and anxiety. Aromas such as lavender, mint and chamomile are very relaxing. Every person has a scent profile that they might find more calming than another. Combine one or more aromas by way of candles or oils and sit in a comfortable area with assured peace and quiet. This is very soothing. You'll almost feel the negative energies that cause your stress, anxiety and bad moods begin to leave you. Your spirit will be lighter and there will be an extra spring in your step. Himalayan sea salt also has great homeopathic properties. It takes negative ions from the air around you and cleanses it. A great calming effect is achieved with the use of Himalayan sea salt blocks, candle holders or warmers within your home.

Alternative Options to Traditional Care

Applied Kinesiology

Applied Kinesiology studies our body's muscles and how they function. Testing these muscles through exercise and stretching helps to diagnose structural and muscular difficulties. The use of Applied Kinesiology can help relieve muscle pain, tension or

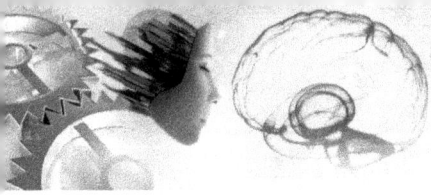

stiffness. Alleviating this pain can help our emotional state. This is due to the fact that muscle aches, stiff joints or other bone/structural pains can actually cause us to feel anger, depression or added stress. All of these factors lead to emotional distress.

There are many other approaches to helping our structural and emotional distresses. The Neural Organization Technique or N.O.T. was developed by Dr. Carl Ferrari. This technique combines several elements to nurture the healing process of both structural and emotional distress simultaneously. Using N.O.T. allows the body to relax and relieve stress by talking through the causes of your stress. Following up with simple chiropractic stretches and structural adjustments can return energy and happy feelings to the body.

Pure Energy techniques such as Reike or Matrix are other options for alternative medicine treatments of emotional, mental and physical distress. Reike was developed in 1922 and was used mainly in Japan for the purpose of stress reduction. Reike is basically the process of lying on your hands to allow 'life force energy' to flow through your bodies. Matrix is defined as the intercellular substance of a tissue or the developing structure of a tissue. The connection between Matrix and emotions is that our emotions are stored in our cells. Using Matrix healing techniques can help those cells to become healthy again.

Acupuncture

Emotions can be held in almost every cell in our bodies. Acupuncturists in Traditional Chinese Medicine actually did correlate emotions to specific organs in the body. Some of those correlations include that fear is related to the kidney, anger is related to the liver and grief is associated with the lungs. Predominantly though, emotions are generally physiologically attached to our brains. The use of acupuncture can help release stored emotions from our spines.

This technique used in Traditional Chinese medicine is still used today and is a highly recommended procedure among alternative medicine specialists for the treatment of stress, muscle aches/pains and overall emotional health.

Chiropractic Care

Chiropractic realignment can be very beneficial to relieving emotional distress as well as muscle, joint or other structural tensions/pains (Chiropractic And The Emotions, 2012). A simple adjustment of our spines releases a lot of pressure and tension, which in turn, releases healthy and happy endorphins, restoring our happy emotions.

Reflexology is a chiropractic technique that applies pressure to our feet, hands or ears by using pressure points to relieve tension. This alternative medicine approach to soothing aches and pains has been proven to work. These sensory parts of our bodies send signals to the brain of relief. The tension is relieved and the stressing or saddening emotions slowly leave our bodies.

All of the techniques mentioned above are used by highly trained Chiropractic Physicians. Alternative medicine approaches to curing emotional disturbances can be much more beneficial than modern day medical practices.

We can benefit from cleansing our bodies of toxins and impurities to maintain a positive flow in our Triangle of Health.

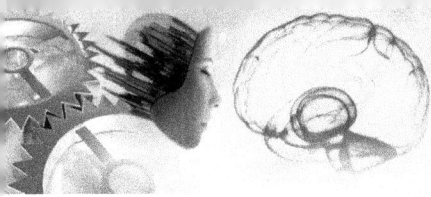

Learning how much our emotional health can interfere with our overall general health may help us to change our lifestyles just a bit in order to achieve total body harmony.

The above techniques will aid in achieving that total body harmony and sound emotional health.

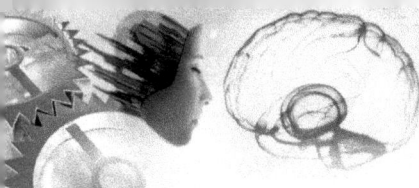

Chapter 4:

Mental State

A healthy mental state comes from taking care of yourself first and foremost. It involves sleeping well, eating right, enjoying yourself and exercising. It also involves loving yourself for who you are. Maintaining proper emotional and physical health are also important to having a healthy and stable mental state. Contributing to life and feeling accomplished, despite setbacks, while setting attainable goals, requires a bit of work on our part. Loving yourself and not punishing yourself for not reaching a goal are healthy mental exercises. Your outlook on life is positive with the realization that not all things will work as planned. Thinking positively about everything isn't the key, the way that you handle a situation is.

Self worth is extremely important for a happy and strong state of mental health. All of us have self-confidence within us and it is up to us to find it and use it when necessary (Jim Pryor 2012). Feelings of inadequacy or failure happen, but finding the positive in a situation and working through it in a constructive manner helps to raise self confidence and self worth. It is natural human nature to use defensive behavior when we feel threatened; nevertheless, doing so in a non-harmful way shows discipline and mental stability. Learning to cope with life's distractions with a positive outcome is a task that is not easily accomplished by all people. Using encouraging thought processes can enable us to move past dark moments. Avoiding life's problems puts them on a shelf in the back of our minds where they are ignored and only enlarge in difficulty. It's best to take each day as it comes, start it with a positive thought and prepare ourselves for what each day might bring. Not accepting failure can be healthy if we tell ourselves that failures along the way led to the ultimate completion of a project or goal.

Feeling mental distress or anguish can happen, sometimes without notice. The way that these feelings are handled will show your mental health capacity. Interpreting and tackling our problems instead of letting them defeat us proves that we have a strong mental state. Not letting feelings of sadness, anger or fear negatively affect us, and assessing the situation causing them is healthy. Dwelling on setbacks or harsh problems is unhealthy. Sometimes we just have to realize that we cannot change the world. We can only change ourselves and how we deal with certain situations that may arise. Being able to function normally and get through each day even when a great loss or traumatic event occurs shows our mental strength. We aren't masking problems; we're simply dealing with them in a productive manner.

The Different Mental States:

The Representational States

A representational mental state means that it stemmed from something. It is a belief that something came from another thing or is associated with one or more items. An example would be that you believe that potatoes are grown in the ground. This is a factual statement, which proves the representation of the thought behind the association. A common confusion is that all representational states come from something being one way only and not accepting that another reason is a possibility. In reality, a thought or idea can stem

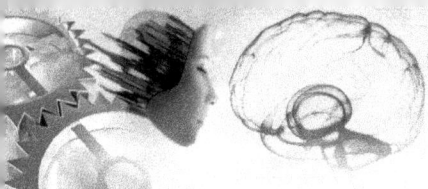

from more than one actual fact or truth. Representational states support a thought or idea that comes from a single belief.

A thought that is represented by a general idea but has an entirely different truth is a propositional attitude. Propositional attitudes are used in two different instances. The first is based on an actual belief that something is true. The second instance is based on wanting or wishing for that instance to occur.

It has long been up for debate that representational states always include or stem from propositional attitudes. On one hand, the two do coincide with each other. On the other hand, they can clash. Arguments easily manifest from one person believing one thing to be true when, in fact, it is completely false. This type of debate can be healthy if the party believing the fact to be true can accept that they are incorrect with proof being provided in a non-aggressive way.

One other mental state to consider as part of the representational states is the intentional state. This mental state describes something being done intentionally, or a thought being expressed with the intent of the reaction being preconceived (Jim Pryor 2012). Keep in mind that there are two different references to intentional states. It is important to be able to correlate between the two when deciding which to use for a specific purpose. Confusion between the two is expected. The intentional state that is included with representational states refers to doing something intentionally. It is simply another term used for representational state.

Qualitative States

In philosophical terms, a qualitative state is defined as a conscious state that may appear to be very different to different people. Two people can experience the same thing and feel it in entirely different ways. This is a conscious state that boggles many minds in its complexity. Many health conditions are categorized by a specific way that someone feels, this is qualitative. The qualitative state refers to someone feeling pain in an individual way. It is difficult to categorize a specific feeling when it comes to using a qualitative state to explain an illness since most people will feel things in slightly different ways from each other.

Perceptual experiences do pair with qualitative states. Perceptual experiences rely heavily on our visual intake of something, or how it looks in reference to something else. Our initial opinion of an object is often defined by our visual perception. Conscious character perception is a major key factor in a qualitative state. Everyone has conscious character, but many of us see things very differently from others. Philosophers often use the terms phenomenal states or phenomenal character. These terms are a more scientific way to explain qualitative states or qualitative character. The phenomena of using our perception to conceive a thought or feeling is categorized as a qualitative state.

There is some controversy as to what qualifies as a representational state and what qualifies as a qualitative state. Both do have similarities within them but have distinct defining factors differentiating between the two. One of the main distinctive differences is that there is no one specific way that someone can feel about a belief. Not all representational states

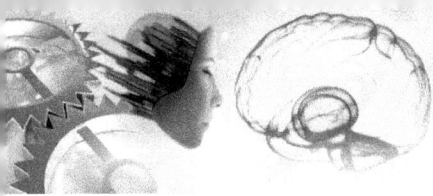

are considered to be qualitative; the previous sentence distinguishes an example of this directly.

Conflict between Philosophers regarding representational and qualitative states distinguishes that they do not believe that there is a similarity between the two. Proven thought process studies show differently. What causes the most debate is that some Philosophers agree that perceptual states are considered to be representational states while qualitative states cannot correlate. The fact of the matter is that, in both respects, both sides are correct. Bodily sensations and pains are felt in different ways, thus representing a qualitative state (Mental States, 2012). These are not generally categorized as a representational state due to the fact that these are conscious feelings stemming from a result.

Not to contradict any previous statements, many representational and qualitative states can be deemed as interchangeable. In many aspects these two mental states do overlap with various similarities. The debate distinguishing these mental states as 'similar' or 'entirely different' will remain, as the situation is not a clear cut regarding either of them. Both derive from general realizations based on facts and beliefs.

Overview of Mental Disorders

Mental disorders often stem from chemical imbalance issues within the brain. It is common for a person to suffer from more than one mental disorder as some are related. The basis of one disorder may be the cause of another, connecting them together. Mental disorders can easily incapacitate a person.

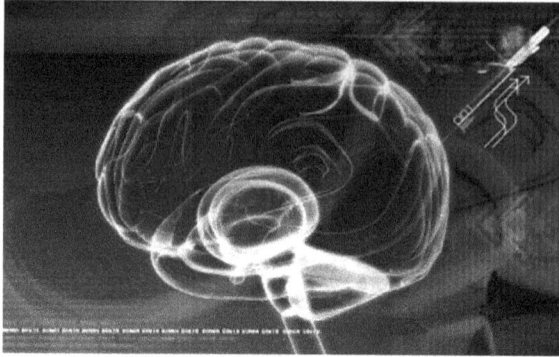

A person's actions or decisions are alteres by the inability of the brain to process thoughts and actions properly. Their ability or inability to function in a 'normal' fashion is determined by their ability to comprehend, act and react to theoretical situations. A mental disorder has a severe impact on a person's general well-being.

Psychiatric disorders of varying severity can group together to compile into one mental disorder. Psychological inadequacies also play a part in defining a mental disorder or psychiatric disorder. An abundance of deciding factors play a role in the determination of a specific disorder. Some of these elements include genetics, learned behavior, physical health, personality, coping skills and previous physiological experiences.

The Diagnostic and Statistical Manual of Mental Disorders, Fourth Edition, or DSMIV, is a compilation by the American Psychiatric Association. It is a detailed book categorizing the different mental illnesses. This manual is updated quite often to remain current. In this manual, it is explained that many mental illnesses are treatable. It is also outlined that people suffering from mental illness can still lead a normal and productive life

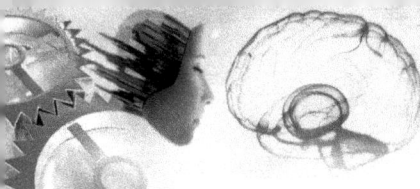

without complication as long as their treatment and/or medication plan is followed properly.

Psychotic Disorders

People who suffer from psychotic disorders are categorized as having the inability to rationally or reasonably process their thoughts or actions. Irrational thought processes can cause such symptoms as confusion, irritability, rage, psychotic tendencies or delusional thoughts. In some cases, hallucinations may occur. A person who is suffering from a psychotic disorder experiences thoughts that are jumbled and which may appear very abstract. To them, this is normal, but for others observing this behavior, it is erratic or abnormal behavior.

The main Psychotic Disorders are Schizophrenia, Schizoaffective Disorder and a group of delusional disorders. Schizophrenia is a very severe disorder that does require therapy and medication to maintain a 'normal' functionality. Schizophrenics suffer from delusional thoughts, hallucinations and general agitation. Social withdrawal and apathy are also common symptoms of Schizophrenia.

Schizoaffective Disorder is a complex disorder that combines Schizophrenia and affective illness. The onset of symptoms mostly follow a significantly stressful situation. This is often more treatable and has a better prognosis than general Schizophrenia.

Mood Disorders

Mood disorders are characterized by disturbances in the general emotional state and the mood of a person's psyche. Mood disorders affect how a person acts, thinks and perceives

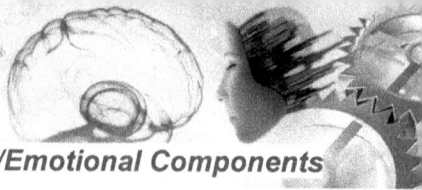

the environment around them. Depression, or an overwhelming feeling of sadness, is the leading factor in diagnosing a mood disorder. Mania, or a roller coaster of emotion, is another defining factor. Bipolar disorder is a mood disorder (Mental States, 2012) in which a person will suffer from alternating bouts of depression and mania. Bipolar disorder must be controlled with a strict regimen of prescription medication and psycho-therapy.

Eating Disorders

Anorexia Nervosa and Bulimia Nervosa are the two main eating disorders. An eating disorder is described as a noticeable disturbance in eating behavior. A person suffering from Anorexia sees themselves as overweight and refuses to eat. They feel guilt for eating and fear that a tiny bite of food will cause a significant amount of weight gain. Their view of themselves is very impaired and delusional. Anorexia mainly affects young women and is very rare in men. Women's perceptions of themselves are dictated by society and what is considered to be acceptable or attractive. There are four main criteria that classify a person as Anorexic. The first is that a patient remains at least 15% under their normal expected body weight and fails to maintain proper weight gain for their age and frame. The second is that the person has an overall fear of gaining weight or becoming obese. Thirdly, one has disturbances in the way that they view their body shape, size or dimensions. Lastly, Amenorrhea, the absence of at least three menstrual cycles in a consecutive period of time, takes place. Lack of nutrition and proper body maintenance can cause this to happen.

Bulimia Nervosa is a disorder in which a person will binge eat and purge following their consumption of food.

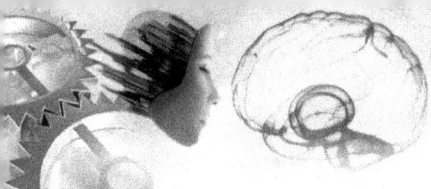

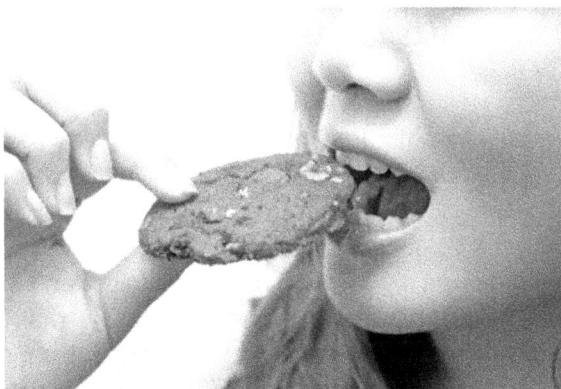

Guilt comes into play almost immediately after consuming food. Those that suffer from Bulimia often feel that they do not have any control over the amount of food that they are eating. They often eat more than others, or more than what is considered to be normal, and feel a sense of regret later. The act of compensating and binging usually occurs two to three times per week with the recurrence or continuance of the pattern lasting for at least three months. Bulimia Nervosa sufferers use such measures as vomiting, using laxatives and diuretics, excessive exercise, fasting or the use of an enema to rid their bodies of calories or foods that they believe could cause excessive weight gain. It is common for a Bulimic person to binge or purge in private. They often feel shame for what they are feeling and/or experiencing with the disorder.

Eating disorders are mental disorders where the mind of an individual changes their perception of themselves. The people with these disorders see themselves as undesirable, unattractive or obese. Denial is often one of the first defense mechanisms noticed when a person suffering from one of these disorders is confronted.

Substance Use Disorders

The use of some substances can form dependency issues. These issues can be a lack of performance at work or school, violent or criminal tendencies, absenteeism, intoxication or accidents. These happenings occur from the substance having a reaction with the central nervous system. The group that is most commonly affected by this problem is adolescents. Men are more susceptible to substance abuse problems than women. Often enough, emotional issues or prolonged substance abuse leads to stronger drug use such as cocaine, heroin or alcoholism (Mental States, 2012). Substance abuse coupled with alcoholism can lead to other behavioral disorders such as, persistent amnestic disorder, Wernicke's encephalopathy and Korsakoff's syndrome.

Somatoform Disorders

Somatoform disorders are summarized as a patient's disbelief in a doctor's diagnosis. With this disorder, a patient will believe that something more is wrong with them and will seek out the medical advice of several professionals. Thoughts of inadequate healthcare cause a person suffering from this disorder to persistently seek medical attention with the same complaints wanting a different result. In most cases, all of the symptoms being experienced are downgraded and not fully explained during an examination. Women are more likely, at 1.5% of the general population, to suffer from this disorder than men, at a rate of 0.2%. Complete remission from this disorder is a rarity. It often originates in the teenage years of life, and for women, shortly after the onset of menstruation. Anyone that may suffer from this disorder will have apparent symptoms by age 25. Related disorders to Somatoform Disorders include antisocial

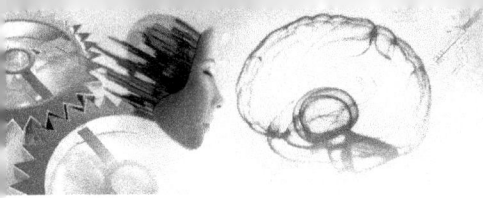

personality disorder, most commonly seen in men, and Dyspareunia or painful sexual intercourse, that is seen predominantly in women.

Personality Disorders

Personality disorders are often detected in adolescents. They are categorized as deeply ingrained, maladaptive patterns of behavior. In some cases, the symptoms remain throughout adulthood. Personality disorders affect an individual and society as a whole. Some personality disorders are genetic; others are triggered by injury or severe trauma. Physicians often have a difficult time diagnosing personality disorders correctly due to their complexity.

The most commonly recognized symptoms are social disconnection, delusions of grandeur, impulsive behavior, irritability, attention craving, dishonesty and aggressiveness. Malnutrition, poor personal care and hygiene, self destruction and a complete retracting from society are severe indications that a personality disorder is occurring.

Anxiety Disorders

Anxiety Disorders combine both mental and physical manifestations of anxiety that do not stem from actual danger. It can be disguised well but is seen as a sudden attack or persistent issue. Attacks are called Panic Disorder while the prolonged or persistent form is called Generalized Anxiety Disorder. The symptoms include fear, anxious thoughts and increased heart rate. These symptoms occur due to a stimulation of the autonomic nervous system. The family of Anxiety Disorders includes Post-Traumatic Stress Syndrome,

Obsessive-Compulsive Disorder and Phobias including social phobia.

Dissociative Disorders

Dissociative disorders are easily explained as an inability to remember important personal information. Ordinary forgetfulness is too light a term to illustrate this disorder. The extremely complicated symptoms include sudden changes in consciousness, identity, motor skills, thoughts, feelings and the perception of reality. Patients will suffer three main similarities though; these include disphoria, suffering and maladaptive functioning. The family of dissociative disorders includes amnesia, dissociative identity disorder, depersonalization disorder and other dissociative disorders.

Impulse Control Disorders

Sufferers of Impulse Control Disorders are unable to resist temptation or unable to act on impulse. Rational decisions are difficult to make. In extreme cases, it is the inability to resist self harm. Impulse control disorders can also be directed toward a person's inability to resist hurting another without rational thought. The most recognizable disorders in this group are Kleptomania, Pyromania, Compulsive shopping, compulsive Gambling and Trichotillomania. Trichotillomania is the irresistible urge to pull out one's own hair.

Symptoms and Biology of Mental Disorders

Noticeable signs and symptoms of mental illness vary greatly. Each disorder does have defining characteristics, but can often

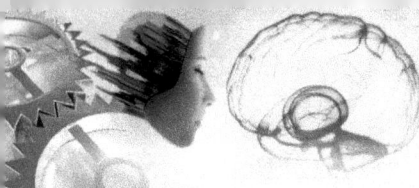

be paired with a combination of other non-stereotypical symptoms as well. Some people suffer from a multitude of mental disorders. Emotions, thoughts and behaviors can all be affected by mental illness. These symptoms can take over a person's life, making it impossible for them to function. One's thought processes, emotions and overall physical health can be affected. People should be observant for radical changes in their mood, emotional or mental incapacity, overall function, eating habits, sleeping habits and other general mental capacity functions. Some symptoms of mental disorders also include chest pain, fatigue, back pain, weight gain, sweating, social withdrawal, dizziness, illicit drug usage, alcoholism, digestive problems, dry mouth, delusional thoughts, erratic behaviors and hallucinations (Chiropractic in Mental Ailments, 2012). If you, a family member or person that you know may be suffering from a mental disorder, it is best to seek the help of a Physician or Psychological expert.

Causes and Risk Factors for Mental Disorders and Illnesses

There is not a defined explanation of what exactly causes mental illness. Definitions are based upon beliefs and observations. Correlations are fused together by studying the behavioral patterns and the general biology of the brain to make these determinations. The search for an explanation continues as scientists strive to cure mental illness.

The biology of mental disorders is difficult to rationalize. Scientists have a difficult time ascertaining what causes them to happen, other than a chemical imbalance in the brain. The causes of the imbalance are not completely clear. The general consensus amongst scientists is that a disconnection or communication error happens within the neurons in the brain. An example of this is that people suffering from depression have a lower amount of the neurotransmitter serotonin. Scientists also believe that those suffering from Schizophrenia suffer from a lack of the neurotransmitters dopamine, glutamate and norepinephrine. The exact biology of mental illness has yet to be deciphered, and findings are merely beliefs based upon studies of individuals that suffer from mental disorders and mental illness. Although the actual cause of mental illness cannot be defined, the risk factors of development have been characterized. Some of these risk factors are genetic while others are social or environmental. An example of this would be a person's genes determining whether they are at risk for Autism, Bipolar Disorder, ADHD or Schizophrenia. The general belief amongst scientists is that more than one gene must be affected to cause a mental illness or disorder and find it unlikely that a single gene anomaly would cause such detriment to the human brain. Statistics about Mental Illness

It is estimated that 1 in 100 people in the world suffer from a Mental Illness. If these people receive the proper medical care, they can function normally, often without any symptoms showing. Some of the world's statistics regarding mental illness are shocking. Suicide is at an astonishing rate of 16% of the world's population. This rate is higher in the United States at about 11 people per 100,000 and in the UK it is much lower at 6 per 100,000 (Identifying mental state, 2012). A surprising 80 million work days are lost by employees each year due to depression and/or anxiety disorders. In the United States, 5.7 million people in the US suffer from bipolar disorder. It is also estimated that over 70% of the prison population suffers from one or more mental disorders. Studies show that 1 in 10

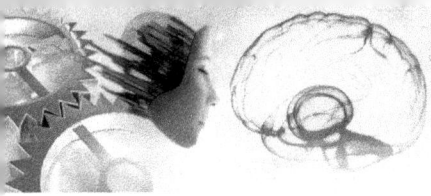

children are diagnosed with a mental illness before the age of 15. In the US, those on Social Security Disability take up four out of ten cases. Mental illness is much more common than one might think and affects about one in five families.

Treatment for Mental Illness

There are multitudes of mental illness medications available to help treat many of these disorders. Some general treatment options available are anti-depressants, mood stabilizers, anti-anxiety medication, anti-psychotic medication and Psychotherapy. Alternative medical treatment options seem to be generating substantially more interest. One example is brain stimulation therapy used to treat depression. Some cases of mental illness are so severe and require hospitalization. This is determined when the sufferer is an immediate threat to themselves or someone else and must be monitored at all times.

Chinese medicine is gaining popularity in the world of alternative medicine for treating mental health problems. Acupuncture and herbal remedies have been used long before the 21st Century in China to treat these illnesses. In the early 19th Century, documentations were made regarding the use of herbal remedies helping ailing mental illness patients to some extent. After the Opium War, millions turned to Fog Tea of Tiamnu Mountain for curing an addiction to opium. Many physicians and health officials, however, remain skeptical about the fact that alternative medicine can help cure a person's mental illness. In addition to natural medicine, self discipline is required, but just sticking to the suggested regimen can also be of great assistance to anyone suffering from a mental illness. Alternative treatment options, such as herbal treatments, can help stimulate normal function within the brain. This can alleviate some of the symptoms experienced by sufferers.

Western medicinal practices may also lead one to a Chiropractor's office. Chiropractors practicing western medicine do not promote the use of prescription medications for many ailments. It is believed that a treatment plan of talk therapy, nutrition and acupuncture therapy will heal physical pain.

Nutritional supplements can help with the stabilization of those suffering from disorders such as bipolar disorder, severe depression, obsessive-compulsive disorder and schizophrenia. Nutritional supplements do not come with the severe side effects that man-made pharmaceuticals can. Lithium is a medication prescribed by traditional doctors to treat bipolar disorder (Infinite Minds, 2012). Some of the side effects associated with Lithium are weight gain, hair loss, memory impairment, hand tremors and decreased thyroid function. Previous studies show that the lack of certain vitamins, minerals and nutrients actually contributes to the risk of developing a mental disorder or mental illness.

Alternative medicine and nutrition therapy can be beyond beneficial in treating mental disorders. A person's overall physical health is often the basis of their overall mental health. Using alternative medicine also reduces the risk of substance dependency. Many of the treatment options and their success are proven to work. It is very important to remember that alternative medicine, western medicine and other natural treatment options will not work for every mental illness patient. The severity of a person's symptoms or condition determines the course of action that is best suited for the individual.

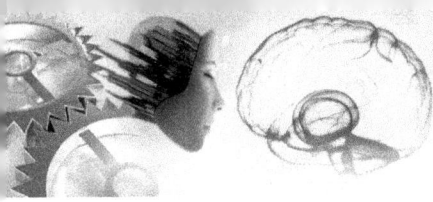

Chapter 5:

Rest versus Sleep

There are many ways people view sleep and rest. They can be used at different times to mean different things. Rest is a state where the body is inactive. The person often lies down or lounges in a still setting allowing the body to rejuvenate (The difference between rest and sleep, 2012). An example of rest is if a person lies on the couch to watch television. This resting is good to do from time to time especially if the body is extremely active. Sleep is a different concept altogether. Sleep occurs when the body shuts down completely.. Often, the heart rate slows down and the body enters the REM cycle. REM is rapid eye movement, or dream state and the longest lasting cycle. This is when the body is asleep.

When one is ready to go to sleep, they first need to let the body rest and relax. Some people can rest and feel good while others need to actually sleep to feel good. A person who is just resting is still alert and their body functions are not delayed. A person who is asleep has a slower reaction time as their functions have slowed down tremendously. The two different states have a common goal to provide relaxation and rejuvenation. Body functions are slower in each state. Although just resting can be beneficial, the body still needs a certain amount of actual sleep to recharge the body. The body regenerates and lets the muscles have a break from doing work to be ready for the next day. Most people are able to get a decent night's sleep but there are factors that cause them to wake before they intended to. Some of these forces are restless leg syndrome, nightmares, insomnia and bed-wetting. All of these are physical (except nightmares) and can be fixed with medical help.

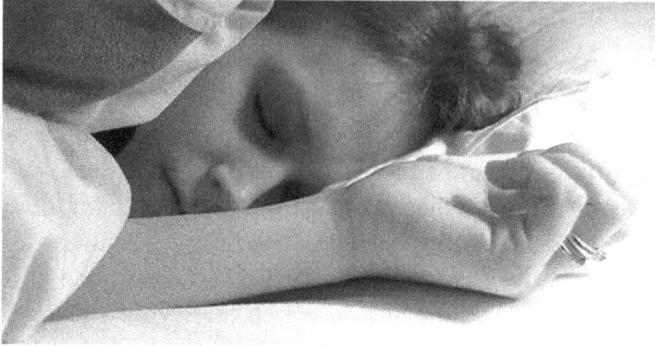

Physiology of sleep

The main goal of this section is to help people understand the difference between sleep and rest. Scientists and philosophers have thought sleep is a type of passive, unconscious state of being. They have found through research, however, that during sleep the brain retains some of its activities. It reacts to internal stimuli rather than external stimuli. The general definition of sleep is: the state of unconsciousness from which a person can be aroused. It also is said that the brain is active at some stages. The exact function of sleep is unknown. However, it is a critical state each living organism needs to experience to function. Although the patterns are different, each living organism needs sleep.

The states of being awake and sleeping are both triggered by neurons. These neurons can be manipulated by things such as alcohol, tobacco, legal and illegal drugs. When an alcoholic is going through withdrawals or drinking heavily, they may not be able to fall asleep. When they do, their REM cycle is erratic and

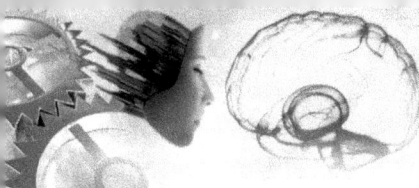

they do not get a full night's sleep. Due to certain medical conditions, taking prescription drugs cannot be avoided, in which case the person can request an alternative medication to help their sleep issue.

Stages of Sleep

An EEG or Electroencephalogram is a type of monitoring system for the brain. This device picks up neurons through their electrical impulses. There are electrodes that are attached to the subject's scalp to record information. A person who is awake has more neuron activity than a person who is asleep. Such research has enabled scientists to place sleep patterns in five categories. The patterns on a person who is awake are rapid and the neurons fire at irregular intervals. They fire at different strengths, making a scattered pattern. One example to show this would be a person standing in a crowded, noisy room. The person can hear a number of voices but cannot pick out just one voice to focus on. This irregular activity is called beta waves. When a person is just at a restful state, the waves would be called alpha waves and move at a slower rate. Although alpha waves may show some irregularity, they are actually smooth and organized waves. The five stages talked about earlier are one through four of non REM sleep and REM sleep. Once the final stage is reached, the cycle goes backwards through the five stages waking the body up. If at any time any of the stages are interrupted by an outside force, the cycle will stop and the person will have to repeat all the cycles.

Non REM sleep cycles

The Non REM sleep cycle holds the first four stages of sleep. Each of these stages can last anywhere from five minutes to 15

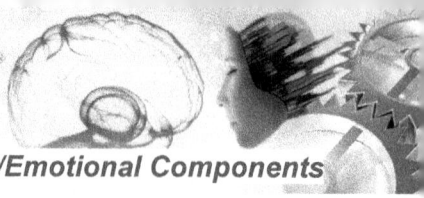

minutes of sleep. The fifth stage cannot be reached if the first four stages do not occur. A sleep study will show a lack of activity in the early stages. In this stage, the eyes are often closed and the person may be aroused without difficulty. If the person is aroused during this stage, they may feel as if they had not slept at all when actually, they were asleep for five to ten minutes. Some people experience a feeling of falling and may cause the body to jump or twitch. This twitching is called hypnic myoclonia. The second stage sleep study will show valleys and peaks in the reading. The waves show periods of muscle relation with spontaneous muscle movement. During this stage, the body temperature and heart rate both decrease. At this point, the body is preparing for the third and fourth stages of deep sleep. The fourth stage is a deeper sleep than the third stage. These stages are often called delta or slow-wave sleep. If a person is woken up during either stage, they will feel a sense of disorientation. During the first four stages of sleep, the body strengthens the immune system and builds muscle and tissue. It is a regeneration period. Studies show that as a person ages they sleep lighter and get less sleep. Their bodies do not require the same amount of sleep as a child or a teenager does. Most elderly people sleep less than 7 hours each night.

REM Sleep

The fifth and final sleep stage is called REM stage. This stage often occurs within 90 minutes of falling asleep. During the first cycle, this period of lasts about 10 minutes and becomes longer with each cycle the final cycle can last up to an hour. Sleep study patterns show that brain waves in this state look similar to those that occur when a person is awake. The person's breathing and heart rate speed up and their eyes move back and forth. During this period extreme brain activity causes

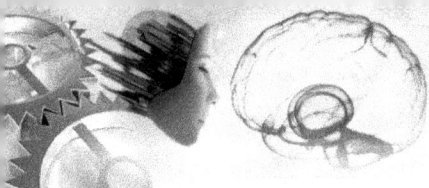

dreams to occur. This activity, called paradoxical sleep, is a mix of brain waves and muscle movements. This type of sleep is more common in infants and childhood. As a person ages, this "dream cycle" will diminish tremendously. Infants spend 50% of their time in this cycle, teens spend about 30%, and adults spend 20%.

Amount of Sleep Required

The amount of sleep a person needs varies from individual to individual. One of the factors determining the amount of sleep a person may need is their age. It is said that an infant will need between 16 and 18 hours of sleep each day. A teen will usually require around nine and an adult can get by on at least seven to eight hours. The amount of sleep needed will increase if the person has not slept very well recently. Not getting the sleep the body needs will result in impaired memory and depression. Some people often get sick because their immune system has not had a chance to regenerate. Also, not getting enough sleep increases the perception of pain. Some people will take caffeine or drink coffee to override the effects of feeling tired. This will only temporarily take care of the problem. After the caffeine effect wears off the person may find himself or herself more tired than they were before they drank the caffeine. Therefore, caffeine is only a temporary fix that the person may become addicted to if they are not careful.

Sleep issues in the USA

We discussed before that sleep cycles are divided into five stages, four non-REM stages and the REM stage. Stage one of the cycle is the lightest sleep when one can be aroused easily. Stage four is the deepest and it will take some time to arouse a person at this stage. If one's cycle is repeatedly interrupted they will not be able to get a good night's sleep. The person will feel tired and sluggish all day long. They will have problems with paying attention and retaining information while they are awake. These people pose a greater risks of causing an auto or some other type of accident, perhaps while at work. There are disorders that cause lack of sleep in America. Some of these disorders are Circadian Rhythm Disorder, Insomnia, Snoring, Nightmares, Restless leg syndrome, sleepwalking and Night terrors.

Circadian Rhythm Disorder

Most people are able to do their sleeping at night because most people have a job that is from 9-5. This sleep is a natural rhythm that the body has created. It could also be described as our internal clock. It is a small part of the brain located in the hypothalamus. It sits above the nerves near the back of the eyes. Exercise and light can reset this brain clock and can move it backwards and forwards. Abnormalities of this clock are known as the Circadian Rhythm Disorder. This type of disorder includes things such as jet lag, new shifts at work, or delayed sleep phase syndrome, when a person falls asleep and wakes up too late or too early. Many people in the world suffer from this type of disorder.

Insomnia

There are many people who struggle with insomnia. They feel that they are not getting enough sleep at night. They struggle to fall asleep and have trouble staying asleep the majority of the time. They may wake up with every little sound because they are not going through the stages of sleep.

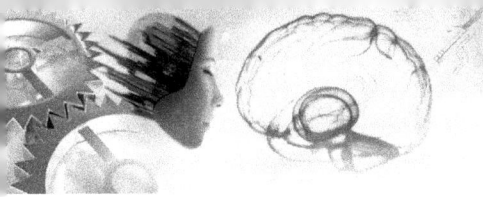

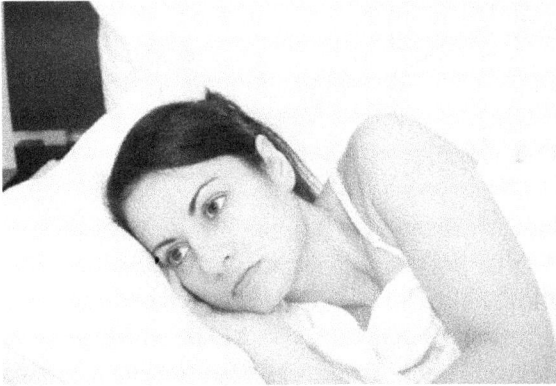

There are many causes for insomnia including jet lag, anxiety, depression, stress, or taking medications. Insomnia may be a temporary occurrence. If a person is a frequent traveler and jumps many time zones, they may have trouble sleeping. In addition, if the person is a coffee drinker this may affect their sleep pattern. There are many medications that people take that may cause them not to be able to sleep. They should consult with their doctor before taking any type of medication. Insomnia will affect a person's daily activity. They may be drowsy or irritable. Insomnia may become a long-term issue if the person does not seek help for this disorder. There is at least one time in each person's life where they will experience a bout of insomnia that can be attributed to many factors.

Snoring

There is at least one person who snores in each household. A snore is produced when air rattles over the relaxed tissue of the throat. Snoring may lead to sleep apnea when the person stops breathing for a short period of time during sleep. The body has to struggle to get going again causing the person to become exhausted. Snoring is caused by things such as allergies, asthma or colds. And is more common in those who are overweight. Snoring may also be an issue for people who cannot tune it out causing them not to get good night's sleep.

Sleep Apnea

Sleep apnea is caused by the upper airway becoming blocked. It interrupts the normal breathing pattern of the person. The person often wakes up struggling to catch their breath. This will also interrupt the sleep cycles and make the person extremely sleepy during the day. This type of disorder, if left untreated, may cause high blood pressure, heart attack or stroke. This disorder is found mostly in overweight older men. However, this abnormal breathing pattern can affect people of any sex and age. About 30% of the people with this issue are not overweight. The person who suffers from this disorder often has a more narrow throat. The person also has a drop in blood oxygen levels during the Apnea. The body is awakened when it is agitated trying to get the air it needs. A person with this disorder should avoid drinking alcohol because it relaxes the muscles even more. A rare apnea disorder occurs when a signal from the brain decreases the muscle strength in the throat. A person who has this type of apnea may not snore. There are breathing machines that a person with sleep apnea can wear that deliver constant oxygen to the body through the nose.

Sleeping and Pregnancy

Women often have trouble in sleeping when they are pregnant, especially when they are further along in their pregnancy. During the first part of the woman's pregnancy, she will be woken up by more trips to the restroom as well as morning sickness. In the latter stages of pregnancy, she will have dreams

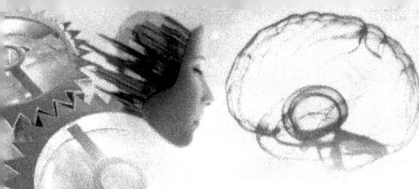

of the baby and discomfort from the baby being so large in her womb. In addition, after the baby is born, the mother may experience issues of having to frequently get up with the baby and postpartum depression. During the first trimester, the mother will have hormonal changes, which may also effect her sleeping. A woman may also be too excited to sleep anticipating her new arrival. Sleep apnea may occur with the woman when she is pregnant due to her ever-changing body. The blood oxygen often drops as the baby is taking most of the mother's nutrients. She will struggle finding a good position to sleep in. Doctors often say pregnant women should sleep on their left side to avoid squishing the artery in the middle of their chest that may be affected if they sleep on their right side.

Narcolepsy

Another common disorder is called narcolepsy. Narcolepsy is a brain disorder that causes a person to be exhausted during the day. Sometimes this can be genetic, but most will report they have no family link to the issue. Sometimes these people will experience "sleep attacks", when they can fall asleep very easily. Most however, suffer from extreme tiredness during the day hours. Some rare nerve disorders may be associated with narcolepsy and it can be diagnosed by performing a sleep study on the patient.

Restless Leg Syndrome

Restless leg Syndrome or RLS is caused when somebody has discomfort and tingling peaks in their legs and feet during the evening and night. The person feels the need to move their legs around to get relief. They may kick their legs or move them as if they are cycling a bike. This movement may cause them to interrupt their sleep cycle and wake up periodically. This is usually more common among older and middle aged adults. Some possible causes of this disorder are kidney failure, nerve disorders, iron or other vitamin deficiency, pregnancy and some types of medications such as antidepressants. It is reported that about 50% of people have a relative with the same issues. There is medication on the market that can be prescribed by a doctor that will help with this issue.

Nightmares

Nightmares occur during the fifth and final stage of sleep. This is the REM cycle. The person will have increased breathing and rapid eye movement. They will most often be so frightened they are awakened from this. There is no scientific cause to nightmares. They can be caused by stress, fever or illness. Most nightmares occur in younger children. It is often dealing with being lost or something that they have seen on TV. Adults rarely have nightmares but when they do, they are often caused by stress.

Night Terrors and Sleepwalking

Sleepwalking and night terrors both occur during the non-REM cycles. They occur in children between the ages of 3 to 5 years. A night terror is dramatic for the child. They will wake up screaming but not be able to explain why they are afraid. Sometimes they will remember seeing something that frightened them but most do not remember a thing. Night terrors are more frightening for the parent than for the child. Sleepwalking can often be dangerous when the person leaves the house or even drives. Sleepwalking can be caused by age or by medication. A night terror can occasionally affect an adult if

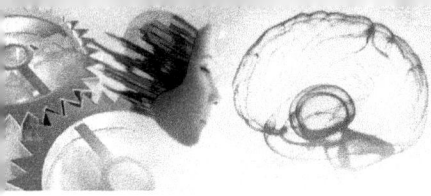

they are having emotional issues or are on medications. Many medications that cause sleepwalking will have a warning on the label. If a person notices such a warning or is told they are sleep walking while on the medication, they should stop taking it immediately and contact their doctor for an alternative measure to their medical issue.

Some factors that affect sleep may be medication, age, lifestyle and health problems. Children usually sleep between ten and fourteen hours per day and their sleep is deeper than that of adults. People who drink a lot of caffeine or smoke will have a harder time falling asleep. There are medications that often cause a person to be sleepy during the day and awake at night. The medications often cause the person to feel anxious or too depressed to sleep. Some common health problems that cause insomnia are lung and heart failure.

Insufficient sleep: a Public Health Issue

Sleep is undoubtedly crucial to a person's health. Insufficient sleep has caused many car accidents. It has also been linked to many accidents in the work place, industrial and medical. Nodding off while driving or not having a clear head will cause these issues. Some people who do not get enough sleep will often suffer from diseases such as hypertension, diabetes, depression and obesity. They are also more likely to get cancer and die at a younger age. There are many factors contributing to a lack of sleep, such as work schedule, societal issues and physical ailments. It is estimated in the United States that 50-70 million adults suffer from a sleep disorder, snoring being the most common. The CDC and the National Center on Sleep Disorders want to keep an adequate surveillance on the sleep habits of the US population due to the increase of sleep deprivation among Americans. Studies are done every so often to monitor sleep patterns of the population, with results usually broken down by sex and age.

Sleep-Related Unhealthy Behaviors

The behavioral Risk Factor Surveillance System, or BRFSS for short, showed a problem regarding the perceived insufficiency of sleep in the year 2008. The last study occurred in the year 1995. They did a four-question model showing that 74,571 adults said they got less than 7 hours of sleep per night. They said this was due to snoring or falling asleep during the day and not getting to sleep at night. The study also showed a staggering amount of people admitting they have dozed off while driving. They have estimated that drowsy driving has been responsible for 1,550 deaths and 40,000 injuries due to vehicle accidents in the United States. There are no official death counts for accidents in the workplace due to nodding off.

Sleep Difficulties Reported by Adults

The National Health and Nutrition Examination Survey, NHANES, did a survey dealing with people's sleeping habits in 2005. The participation was for people of 16 years of age and older. They used data from the years 2005 and 2006 to compile the outcome. There were 10,896 people that responded that were around 20 years of age. The duration of sleep was the most common factor reported at 37%. The report showed that these people were getting less than seven hours of sleep per night. This in turn affected how they functioned during the day. People who are middle aged had an average of about 40%, those that are over 60 were about 32%.

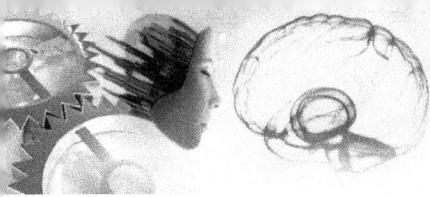

Amount of Sleep Needed Versus Amount Actually Occurring

The need for sleep varies for each person. The amount often changes as the person ages. A school age child generally gets 10 hours of sleep per night. A teenager generally gets about 9 hours and an adult usually gets 7-8 hours each night. About 30% of adults report that they are only getting about 6 hours of sleep per night. Thirty one percent of school age children reported getting 8 hours of sleep in the year 2009. This is due to the increased level of activity the child is involved in. Many students belong to extracurricular activities as well as work a job. They often find themselves doing homework late in the evening and not being able to go to sleep. The student is trying to get too much done during the day and not getting the appropriate amount of rest they need. Usually when they have a day off they will sleep for hours, making their sleep habit more difficult.

Napping Benefits

When people find themselves nodding off or their eyelids too heavy to stay open they need to take a nap. The person is not doing the best they can do. A NASA study showed that a person who took a 40-minute nap recovers at 100%. Another study shows that even a 20-minute "power nap" is beneficial to a person.

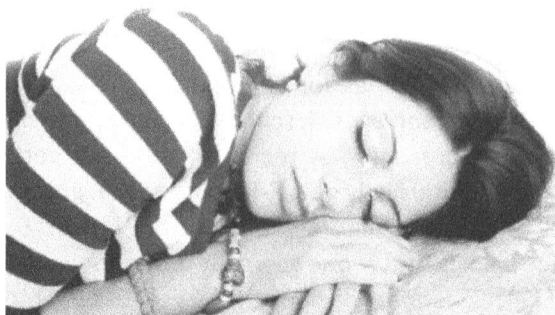

This is better for the body than trying to exercise or taking caffeine. There was also a study conducted to show that pilots who were able to nap for 25 minutes did not nod off like some of their sleep-deprived peers. The pilots who took naps made less errors in taking off and landing. It is a good idea for a person to break up their day with a nap. This will help the person to become more alert for the second half of their day. If the person is going out of town after work, it is best for them to take a nap right before they leave, that way they are refreshed and will be more alert.

Naps also help to improve a person's memory. It will help the person stay focused on the task. The person will be able to multi task better after getting a good nap. This also helps with memory retention. When the person sleeps, the information is transmitted to the neocortex where long-term memories are stored. Many students report studying for a test right before they fall asleep to help retain the information needed to ace the test. Most people refuse to take a nap. They feel they do not have time to be "lazy" during the day. Not taking the time to nap will drastically reduce productivity. The person will be too

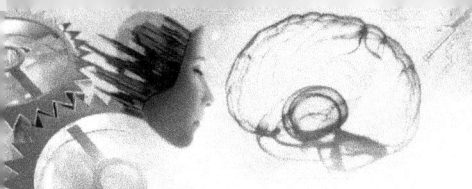

busy yawning and making mistakes instead of getting the job done right the first time.

It is better to take a 30-minute nap to refresh the body and mind. There was a study done for four days on subjects. Those who took naps did better than those who did not. They were able to function better and efficiently complete their task. The ones who did not take the nap struggled and had to do things over, taking more time to do them. Napping also helps sensory perception. It basically means that food will taste better, and things will be more vivid. It also helps increase a person's creativity. It will loosen up the ideas in one's head and allow one to execute them better. Not getting enough sleep will also cause a person to become stressed.

When a person is stressed, the body releases a hormone called cortisol. This hormone helps the body deal with the flight or fight response. It also causes the immune and muscular systems to become weak, causing physical damage to the body. This damage can lead to unwanted disease and sometime early death. When a body is asleep, it releases a growth hormone, which is the antidote to cortisol. It helps reduce stress and ups the person's sexual function. It also is an aid in weight loss. Those that get better sleep at night feel better, function better and live longer.

There is a neurotransmitter called serotonin that helps regulate appetites, mood and sleep. It helps the body stay content and controlled. When a person is stressed, the body blocks the serotonin and the person becomes overwhelmed, depressed and easily distracted. Napping will turn this all around and give the person a more positive outlook even when things seem impossible to accomplish. The perfect nap would be about 90

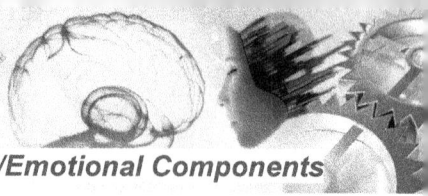

minutes long and is best taken between one and three in the afternoon.

This length of nap will be a good balance to level out each sleep stage. The person needs to tailor their nap to their daily schedule. If possible, the person should try to take their nap at the same time each day that way the body gets on a good schedule. If that is not possible then the person should sleep the same amount of time each day.

Rest and Relaxation

Rest is something that occurs when a person is awake. This can also be called a function of the autonomic nervous system. The ANS also belongs to the peripheral nervous system. It controls many of the body's organs and muscles. Many people do not know about the function of the ANS as it is an involuntary function of the body. For example, people do not notice when a blood vessel changes size within the body. In addition, most people do not notice when their hearts begin to beat faster.

Sometimes all a person has to do is sit down, close their eyes, and relax to continue on with their day. Others need to actually lie down and take a nap. Each person's body is different and each need of the person is different. Rest is good to rehabilitate energy levels. If the person does not get rest, they cannot perform their tasks well and they may fail. Being able to rest depends on how relaxed a person is. If they are tense or have a lot on their mind, they will not be able to rest properly. Instead of resting, some will take caffeine to get their body going. With this, the body will crash and be more tired than it was before when the effect wears off.

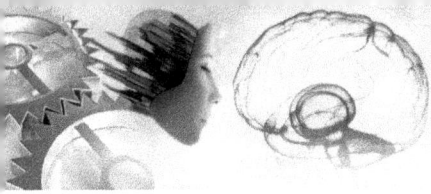

Active and passive Rest

Different types of exercises coincide with different types of rest. Aerobic exercise includes running, cycling or swimming and anaerobic exercise includes lifting weights and yoga Active resting keeps the heart rate up and the body in motion. Passively resting allows the heart rate to drop quickly. Active rest may include things such as briskly walking or jump roping between reps of running.

An example of active rest would be if a person ran on a track for one lap, jogged the next lap, and then repeated. A passive type of rest would be stretching between reps of lifting weights. The person could also walk to catch their breath also exhibiting passive rest. If a person exercises back-to-back, switching things up, different muscle groups are used and some muscles can while still working out others. The person can do an aerobic workout by utilizing an anaerobic one.

This also cuts down on the time for completing the workout. The terms can be used interchangeably with passive and active recovery. An athlete that is determined to do hardcore sets on the track will have a hard time resting. The person believes if they push themselves, that they will become faster and stronger when it actually just makes them tired and they get an insufficient amount of the rest they need to regenerate. This in turn may cause them to become sick or overly tired. Passive rest is when the athlete is not doing anything. This many include things like sleep in between workouts. It can also include days when they lightly work out such as just walking around the track or lifting light weights.

It can also include something that is relaxing like stretching or yoga. The goal of this type of rest is to get the heart rate elevated to increase the blood flow to the muscles. It helps to make sure the muscles do not become stiff or sore. This is a recovery stage for the body after a long, tough workout. When a person is stiff or sore the next day after a workout it is because the cells are damaged. The body will set to work to repair these damaged cells. If the athlete allows it, the body will eventually repair the damaged cells completely.

If the athlete does not give the body adequate time to rest and repair they will start their next workout in a weakened state and may further damage cells. If he continues this spiral downwards, he will become fatigued and have difficulty sleeping, eating and retaining information. This is called an over trained state. Once this occurs the athlete needs more rest to fix the damage that has been done. The more amount of damage there is, the more rest will be required.

Most athletes think they need to push themselves even harder when they are hurting but this is the wrong way to go about things. They think that if they rest then they will be viewed as weak, but in reality, resting will make them stronger and better able to handle challenges. There are many high school age kids having surgeries from being pushed too hard by their coach. The coach has it in their head that the child is young and in good shape and can handle anything. No matter what the age of a person, everybody needs rest to rejuvenate his or her body.

Different Rest Habits Around the World

European countries have a program where employees can take a month to two month long paid vacation during the year. They call it a "holiday." Some Americans get about four weeks of paid

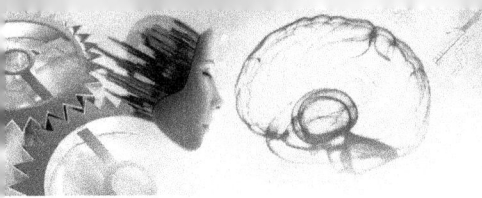

time off per year. In France, the person will get about seven weeks and in Germany, they will get eight weeks. Rest and relaxation is important in order to regenerate and be fresh at work once the person returns.

There was a study done to show that people who live in Europe often work more hours than those that live and work in America. This was done in 1960. A more recent study was done in 2005 to show that Americans increased their work hours while Europeans enjoy their time off.

Today, people in the United States work even more hours than people in Japan. The change is due to the economy and the price of goods going up. The productivity of goods and the worth ethic of America is another reason for the longer work hours. They say that Europeans are more into leisure than other parts of the world. Americans often own bigger cars and bigger houses. They also have vacation homes. It is said that Europeans are not caught up in appearances as Americans are. Americans are usually constantly in contact with the company or checking emails even while on vacation and do not get the rest they need.

In the country of Germany, it is more socially acceptable to take weeks off from work without being interrupted. Europe also has a higher income tax rate than Americans making them less likely to work overtime due to the tax rate. It is also said that Americans will accept less money for more vacation time at a new job. They are being paid less but their hours are increasing, leaving little time for rest and relaxation on a day-to-day basis. Each job is required to give a break depending on the amount of hours the person has worked. If a boss refuses to give a break, the employee can turn them into the HR department or go above their head and report them.

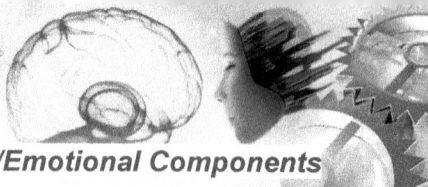

Sleep and Rest Disorder Treatments

A treatment dealing with health that is not in western medical practice is often called alternative medication. A variety of methods is utilized, such as diet and exercise and lifestyle changes, to help issues such as sleep and rest disorders. Some popular treatments for these disorders include: acupuncture, yoga, imagery, hypnosis, aromatherapy, herbal remedies, relaxation and massages. Some treatments for insomnia could be exercise, acupuncture and meditation. Alternative medication is becoming more popular in recent years and is also referred to as the green way or the natural way of living.

Herbal Treatments

There is a root called the Valerian root that has been able to help individuals with sleep disorder. It helps get the person to sleep and keeps them asleep. More studies are needed on this root to conclusively say that it will help people with insomnia (Herbal medicine, 2012). With any herbal treatment, a person should first consult with their doctor or do a bit of research to find if the effects are worth the risk of taking the herb.

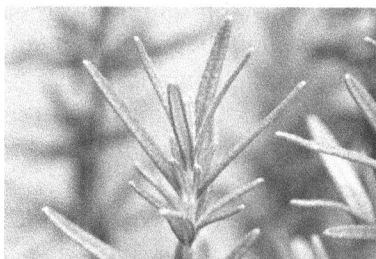

Some other herbal treatments may include chamomile, passionflower, hops, ginseng, lemon balm and skullcap. In the country of Germany, they have approved many of these herbs

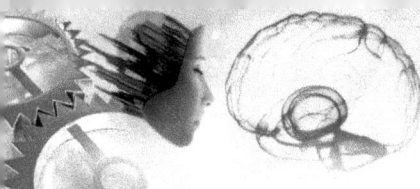

for treatment of insomnia. These herbs are usually a second line of defense when it comes to insomnia. Some herbal medications interact with other medications. A person who would like to take one of these should first consult their doctor to make sure the medication will not mix with the herb causing a bad reaction. Most of these herbal treatments come in a form of a pill that a person takes once, twice and sometimes three times per day. Sometimes these herbs can be used in the form of drops or in a tea to be effective.

Melatonin

Melatonin is a hormone generally found in the brain that stimulates sleep. There is a product that one can take that simulates this hormone (Melatonin and Sleep, 2012). The hormone is located in the pineal gland in the human brain. It can also be found in plants and animals. The effects of melatonin are not completely understood but it does play a critical role in rest and sleep.

Melatonin is often used in treating Circadian Rhythm Disorder discussed earlier. There are minimal adverse effects associated with melatonin. Melatonin is often taken an hour or two before bedtime to initiate a good night's rest. Some parents give this synthetic drug to their children before bed, especially those that are hyperactive and have a hard time falling asleep. It is best to take the most minimal dose of melatonin.

Sleep Disorders and Acupuncture

In traditional Chinese medicine acupuncture is the go-to treatment for insomnia as well as other sleep disorders. This procedure involves using tiny needles that are inserted in various parts of the skin and body. Sometimes this is paired with

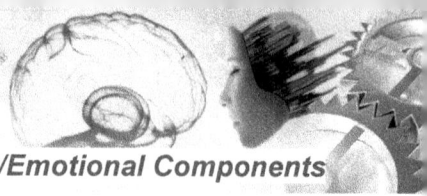

heat or electrical stimulus. The needles are placed to influence certain parts of the body. Studies show that using acupuncture has increased sleep quality in some people with insomnia. More research must be done before we can conclusively say that this is a good treatment. Many places offer acupuncture as an alternative for normal medical treatments. Some women will do acupuncture while in childbirth or do it before hand to stimulate childbirth.

Sleep Disorders Relaxation and Meditation

Muscle tension that increases causes lack of sleep. Therefore, techniques dealing with relaxing the muscles are beneficial and an effective treatment for insomnia. Many people can learn these meditation techniques but it may take them several weeks. They can master them enough to relax their muscles for a better night's rest. It is proven that relaxation in meditation such as Yoga, offers an increase in blood levels of melatonin to regulate sleep. Meditation can be anything from Yoga or deep breathing exercises to become relaxed. Some people enjoy meditation alone in a quiet environment, while others will seek out group meditation in yoga or a meditation retreat.

Sleep Disorder Exercise

When a person gets regular exercise, it deepens their sleep. Even if the person already gets a good amount of regular sleep, exercise will help them regenerate and repair things better while sleeping (Relief From Sleep Disorders by American Chiropractic, 2012). Moderate exercise has been proven to help people sleep better at all ages. The best time to exercise is about three to four hours before bed so the sleep cycle is not

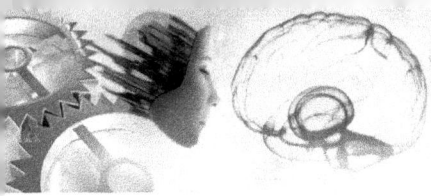

interrupted. Yoga has also been known to help cancer patients sleep better at night. Before a person begins an exercise program, they should first consult with their doctor and let them know the type of routine they will be doing. They need to also be careful not to overextend themselves to keep up with anybody else. They should only do as much as their body can handle.

Alternative Therapy Warnings

Alternative medications are not always safe to take as they may interact with some prescription medications. The first thing to do is to consult a doctor before taking any type of herbal remedy. The person should let the doctor know if they are experiencing adverse reactions such as rapid heartbeat, nausea, vomiting, anxiety, rashes or any other odd feelings. If these reactions are noticed, the person should stop taking the herbal supplement and contact the doctor. When taking herbs, it is best not to take more than one at a time. This may affect the health of the person or the effect of the herb and what it is intended for. The person should only buy branded herbs that show the address, lot and batch number, guidelines and expiration date of the product. It should also list all of the possible side effects of the herb. The person should also purchase these herbs from a reputable business so that the contents and ingredients can be trusted.

Sleep Disorder Chiropractic Medicine

When people are having trouble sleeping the first thing that needs to be done is to make sure it is not due to a physical ailment. This is dealing with the movement of the physical body. Movement is the primary means of survival within the body and it deals with the reptilian brain. Movement is energy in various forms. The body's motion depends on its current position and the surrounding environment.

We live in a time where our bodies are often stressed by the environment around them. There are hundreds of factors such as physical, emotional or electromagnetic factors. When gravity is involved, the skeletal system is extremely important (Relief From Sleep Disorders by American Chiropractic, 2012). Chiropractic care is the best thing for the human frame. Muscles are used to help move the skeletal system. The human body relies on certain patterns to move the body. It also deals with the body's reflexes and Kinesiology. These help to stimulate the patterns or natural reflexes.

People often use Pilates to help balance the core and muscles. Also deep breathing exercises are beneficial to the body, and help to balance the movement of air in and out of the lungs. This helps to balance the respiratory pH of the body. One can also use nutritional treatments to assist in the performing of functions in the body by enabling the body to retain and store these nutrients for future use. Many people wonder how chiropractic care helps in sleep issues such as sleep apnea or insomnia. The body is designed to be able to survive in a hostile environment.

Sometimes an abnormal amount of stress placed on a body will eventually take its toll. It will cause the body's energy reserve to be depleted and the tissue starts to disintegrate. This is the time in a person's life where they feel aches and pains on a daily basis. This may lead to worse pains in the future such as organ dysfunction and structural instability. Holistic Chiropractic care deals with healing of the spinal column and nervous system, aggravated by abnormal stress.

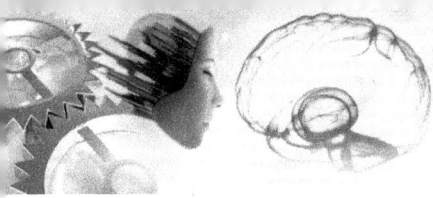

A normal spine and muscles will allow a person to move with no pain and in perfect balance. A Chiropractor's goal is to attempt to restore the stability and balance of the spine, increasing the body's survival ability and adaptability. There is another type of chiropractic care called Chiropractic Neurology. It deals with the brain and central processing unit. The care gathers information that is based on neurological, chiropractic and orthopedic evaluations. Chiropractic Neurology uses rehabilitation and sensory integration tools such as heat, balance, sound and smell. It helps to create an environment for the body to function in. There are many divisions when it comes to chiropractic care.

Chiropractic care helps to restore, repair, build and clear unwanted emotions as well as helping the body detoxify and balance out, allowing a better night's rest. Many people suffer from year to year with ailments, never knowing that all of them can be fixed by visiting a chiropractor. One sign that the spine is off balance is if the person has unusual difficulties breathing.

The next sign is a change in sleep patterns. The person may toss and turn and never be comfortable when trying to sleep. Something that chiropractors have noticed is many people have one shorter leg, often causing loss of balance. There are many places a chiropractor manipulates on the spine to fix these issues. Some people only need a treatment or two per year while others must go a few times per month to get back into a good sleep Habit. Having poor posture opens the body up to many downfalls.

If the person is off balance, they will have more accidents and more aches and pains causing them not to sleep. They will have trouble concentrating and may become depressed, all because their back is "out of whack." Getting regular chiropractic care may be the key to improving a person's sleep habits. The chiropractor may include electrodes to the treatment from time to time.

Sleep Apnea and Snoring

When somebody is snoring or has sleep apnea they are having troubles keeping their head upright due to weakened muscles caused by an imbalance in the spine. These muscles are important to keep the head upright when walking, standing or just sitting still. When the spine is out of place it will put unnecessary pressure on the neck muscles causing severe pain.

Sometimes the neck is stuck at an angle and takes time to heal using chiropractic care and rest. When these muscles are injured they cause postural abnormalities in how the neck reflex works (Snoring and Sleep Apnea, 2012). The muscles that are weak will cause degeneration of the spine, which makes it difficult to sleep and do other activities. An average person moves their body position in bed 25-75 times per night! If the person is having issues, they may not move as much, causing stiffness in the morning, which can affect the rest of their day. The process of turning deals with the muscles of the neck, trunk and arms and legs.

There are four components dealing with this. These are: rolling of the trunk, adduction and abduction of the shoulders, supporting activities of the elbows, and adduction and abduction of the hips. Having poor posture during the night often affects the airflow in and out of the mouth, thus promoting sleep apnea. Having the mouth wide open during sleep causes snoring and blockage associated with sleep apnea and respiratory efforts made by the sleeping person.

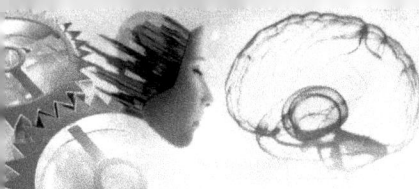

Postural deviation that alters body mechanics puts uneven pressure on the joints that leads to pain and inflammation. The inflammation often sets in and causes biochemical compromises, which often affect the person's motivation and mood. The best thing to do is to try to change the diet at night to help this awkward sleep habit. Many people at this stage are not motivated to try this, however, adding chiropractic and kinesiological treatments will help.

A survey was taken of 500 patients and revealed that patients who have issues with sleep apnea or snoring also have neck and low back pains. A type of exercise to help this is called Pilate. This exercise helps re-educate and tone up the core postural muscles. This will help in reducing inhibitions from a higher center of the brain that cause upper respiratory breathing disorders. This will also lead to increased activation of the muscle fibers causing them not to be able to rest appropriately.

When there is no muscle mass to support the head, the jaw often slips open at night causing sleep apnea and snoring. If stress is left untreated, it will cause fixed stress. Cells and tissue break down resulting in cellular and organic death. There are neurological assessments that can be tested to identify the level of balance in functional components. These tests will also find issues in the left and right hemispheres of the brain. To identify biochemical stability salivary hormones and urinary organic acids need to be tested for PH. A PH level that is out of balance will also affect a sleep pattern.

A person can take medicines to help this or can benefit from chiropractic care. When we commit ourselves to growth and our health, we often recognize that we have to make choices in our life and have the ability to make productive choices. These choices will lead to a healthier and happier life. We will move

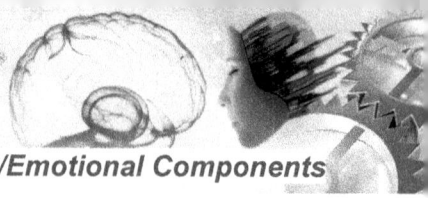

into a perfect pattern easily, showing the greatness of the human design, and its effortless power.

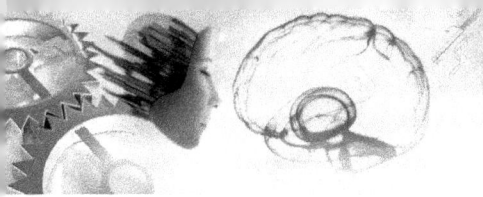

Chapter 6:

Level of Consciousness

The mystery of human consciousness has fascinated scientists for thousands of years. Sir David R. Hawkins, M.D., Ph.D., examines the complex wonders and the many levels of human consciousness in his book, Power vs. Force: "The Hidden Determinants of Human Behavior." Dr. Hawkins proposes there is a scale of consciousness that can be measured. Each level predicts human behavior and beliefs about life and God.

Dr. Hawkins's Scale of Consciousness orders the human consciousness into these levels: shame, guilt, apathy, grief, fear, desire, anger, pride, courage, neutrality, willingness, acceptance, reason, love, joy, peace, enlightenment. The levels are measured by a system developed by Dr. Hawkins that physically tests the muscles. Results are given values from 0 to 1,000. On Dr. Hawkins's scale, shame is the lowest consciousness level, given a vibration value of "20" and enlightenment the highest, given a vibration value of "1,000".

According to Dr. Hawkins, most individuals maintain a steady state of consciousness that can be defined as our "normal" state. People move in and out of the different levels. Dr. Hawkins finds that individuals usually do not vary more than about five points. Some people may vary several hundred points in a lifetime, however.

Dr. Hawkins sets several thresholds of behavior that can be predicted by the level of consciousness. For instance, at vibration levels above 200, self destructive behavior changes to life-enhancing behavior. There are eight vibration levels below 200, the Level of Integrity. According to Speed of Light Films, Dr. Hawkins's levels can be summarized this way:

Shame (20) – Is known as a step ahead of death, this level involves a person contemplating suicide or feelings of wanting to die. This level is also known as a self-destructive phase.

Guilt (30) - This is a step above shame, thoughts of suicide are still being dealt with. The individual still thinks of himself or herself as a sinner and has trouble dealing with things that have happened in the past.

Apathy (50) –This level involves the person feeling victimized or hopeless and is referred to as learned helplessness. This level is common with many homeless people and they are trapped at this level.

Grief (75) -This level often occurs when a person loses a loved one. A sense of loss and sadness in addition to depression is common with grief.

Fear (100) - This level is similar to paranoia, a person thinks that the world is against them or is unsafe for them. It is also comparable to being in an abusive relationship.

Desire (125)- This level can be compared to being materialistic. The person has unimportant desires such as an excess of money, or excessive habits such as smoking, drinking or drug use.

Anger (150) –Anger is known as the level of hatred, a strong dislike for others or things in which he or she may feel are unattainable. It is difficult for a person to come out of this level because it takes more energy.

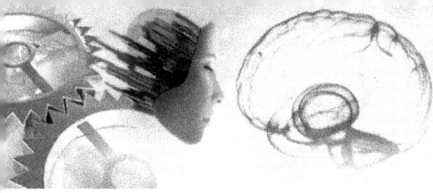

Pride (175) –This level can be misleading, the feeling starts as a good feeling. Unfortunately, the feeling is temporary because it is based on external and artificial occurrences

Dr. Hawkins calibrates the vibration levels on a logarithmic scale, and finds that about 78 percent of the world falls below vibration levels of 200. As one goes higher on the scale, however, their vibration levels counterbalance those below them on an exponential scale. Dr. Hawkins theorizes that one person at level 600 may balance the negative vibrations of about 10 million people below 200.

On Dr. Hawkins's scale, levels between 200 and 700 reflect the evolution of the human consciousness from self-destruction to enlightenment. According to Speed of Light Films, those levels are defined like this:

Courage (200) – This is the first level of true strength where one starts to see life as challenging and exciting instead of overwhelming. This level promotes interest in personal growth, such as skill-building, career advancement, and further education. Here a person starts to see their future as an improvement upon their past, rather than a continuation of the same.

Neutrality (250) - This level is epitomized by the phrase, "live and let live." It's flexible, relaxed, and unattached. Whatever happens, there is no need to have anything to prove. One feels safe and easily relating with other people. This is a very comfortable place sometimes promoting a level of complacency and laziness. Here a person is taking care of their needs, but won't push too hard.

Willingness (310) - At this level a persona is safe and comfortable, and can start using their energy more effectively.

One begins to take action and thinks about time management, productivity, and getting organized, things that weren't so important at the level of neutrality. This is the level where the development of willpower and self-discipline becomes important. This is the point where one's consciousness becomes more organized and disciplined.

Acceptance (350) - This is the level where a powerful shift happens, and one awakens to the possibilities of living proactively. After one becomes competent, their abilities are multiplied to good use. This is the level of setting and achieving goals. This level drives many people to switch careers, start a new business, or change their lifestyle.

Reason (400) - At this level one transcends the emotional aspects of the lower levels and begins to think clearly, rationally, and start making meaningful contributions. Hawkins defines this as the level of medicine and science. At the very high end, this is the level of Einstein and Freud.

Love (500) - Unconditional love, a permanent understanding of one's connectedness with all that exists, a deep sense of compassion. At the level of reason, one is living in service to the mind. At the level of love, one now places their mind and all other talents and abilities in service to one's heart. This is the level of awakening to one's true purpose. All motives at this level are pure and uncorrupted by the desires of the ego. This is the level of lifetime service to humanity and beginning to feel as being guided by a force greater than oneself. Examples are Gandhi, Mother Teresa, and Dr. Albert Schweitzer. Hawkins claims this level is reached only by 1 in 250 people during their entire lifetimes.

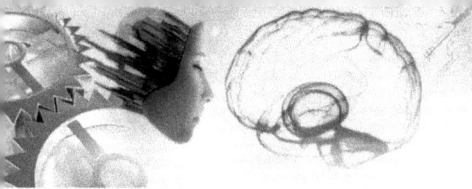

Joy (540) - This is the ultimate state of pervasive, unshakable happiness. Eckhart Tolle describes this state in 'The Power of Now'. This is the level of saints and advanced spiritual teachers. Just being around people at this level makes one feel incredible. At this level life is fully guided by synchronicity and intuition. There's no more need to set goals and make detailed plans — the expansion of your consciousness allows one to operate at a much higher level.

Peace (600) - Supreme transcendence. Hawkins claims this level is reached only by one person in 10 million.

Finally, according to Dr. Hawkins, levels of 700 to 1,000 reflect Enlightenment.   According to Speed of Light Films, the enlightenment levels are defined as:

Enlightenment (700-1000) – This is the highest level of human consciousness, where humanity blends with divinity. It is extremely rare and is the level of Krishna and Buddha. Just thinking and studying about people at this level can raise one's consciousness.

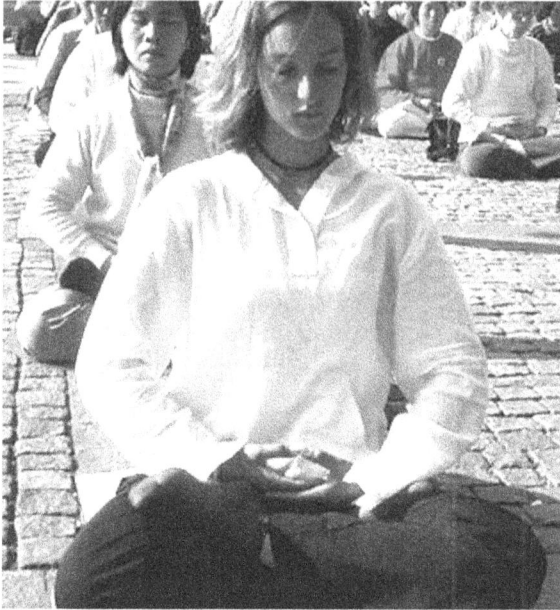

Many individuals find Dr. Hawkins's model worthy of consideration. Dr. Hawkins theorizes that people, events, individual societies, and indeed all of humanity can be effectively evaluated by the measured levels.

People who want to improve their lives can review the levels to determine what level they function in right now. As they progress through life, they can see how they move up and down the scale as they grow. Dr. Hawkins maintains in his book that people operate on several levels simultaneously. One level may predominate in one area of a person's life, while another level is evident in a different area. According to Dr. Hawkins, "An individual's overall level of consciousness is the sum total effect of these various levels."

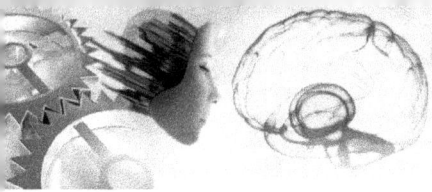

One man, Steve Pavlina, explains his experience this way on his website, Stevepavlina.com:

"One thing I like about these levels of consciousness is that I can trace back over my own life and see how I've been moving through them. I remember being stuck at the level of guilt for a long time – as a child I was indoctrinated into a belief system where I was a helpless sinner, being judged according to the standards of someone at the level of love or higher. From there I graduated to the state of apathy, feeling numb to the whole thing.

By high school I had reached the level of pride — I was a straight-A student, captain of the Academic Decathlon team, showered with accolades and awards, but I became dependent on them. I hit the level of Courage in my late teens, but the courage was very unfocused, and I overdid it and got myself into all sorts of trouble. I then spent about a year in neutrality and moved through willingness and acceptance during my 20s with a lot of conscious effort.

At present I'm at the level of reason and getting closer and closer to completing the leap to love. I experience the state of love more and more often, and it's guiding many of my decisions already, but it hasn't yet stuck as my natural state. I've also experienced the state of joy for days at a time, but never with any permanence yet. That state is a pervasive feeling of natural euphoria, as if I'm exploding on the inside with positive energy. It literally forces me to smile. I've been in that state for most of this morning, probably because I haven't eaten anything yet today (I find it easier to hit that state of consciousness when I eat lightly or not at all) (Steve Pavlina, 2012)."

Referring to the alternation between levels, Pavlina says on his website:

"We'll naturally fluctuate between multiple states throughout the course of any given week, so you'll probably see a range of 3-4 levels where you spend most of your time. One way to figure out your "natural" state is to think about how you perform under pressure. If you squeeze an orange, you get orange juice because that's what's inside. What comes out of you when you get squeezed by external events? Do you become paranoid and shut down (fear)? Do you start yelling at people (anger)? Do you become defensive (pride)? What happens to me under pressure is that I become hyper-analytical, but recently I just had a pressure situation where I handled it mostly by intuition, which was a big change for me. This tells me I'm getting close to the unconditional love state because in that state, intuition can be effectively accessed even under pressure.

Everything in your environment will have an effect on your level of consciousness. TV, Movies, Books, Web sites, People, Places, Objects, Food. If you're at the level of reason, watching TV news (which is predominantly at the levels of fear and desire) will temporarily lower your consciousness. If you're at the level of guilt, TV news will actually raise it up (Steve Pavlina, 2012)."

According to Dr. Hawkins, nearly 85 percent of the world's population has vibration levels under 200. He writes that populations with levels in the low 200s usually are very primitive populations. Those societies are stricken with famine and extreme poverty. Labor is unskilled and housing tends to be temporary.

Societies with levels in the mid-200s have begun crude trading practices, possibly use currency, and have begun to learn to

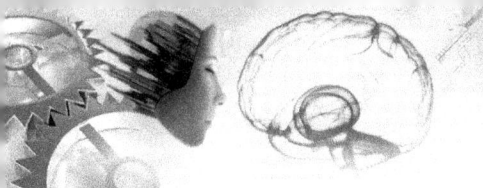

construct permanent housing. Usually there is adequate clothing and food. In these societies, rudimentary education begins.

Civilizations in the high 200's generally are comprised of blue-collar, tradesmen, and retail workers, according to Dr. Hawkins. Fishing has progressed from a necessity in the lower level societies to an industry in this model, he says.

Fear, apathy, and political oppression are common factors in world populations that dwell in Level 200. These difficult circumstances cause people to constantly fight, being pulled down to the point where they are unable to harness the energy to be pulled up.

Dr. Hawkins says in his book that "any meaningful existence cannot even commence until Level 250". At that point, he maintains, some level of self-confidence begins to emerge, and positive life experiences can begin.

According to Dr. Hawkins, after level 200 the next major barrier that people encounter is at vibration levels of 500, the level called "Love'. Dr. Hawkins postulates that love is the beginning of the spiritual world, and many people have difficulty entering that level because they are so rooted in the physical world. Levels in the 400s represent the scientific levels of consciousness. Dr. Hawkins says that the top thinkers of the scientific world, Einstein, Aristotle, and Newton all calibrated at about 499. Because the spiritual realm is formless, many great minds have difficulty making the leap. Dr. Hawkins estimates that only a tiny percentage of the world's population is successful at transcending level 500.

Dr. Hawkins says in his book that for those who progress and reach Peace at Level 600, "nothing is stationary, and all is alive and radiant (Steve Pavlina, 2012)." He goes on to say that at this level people begin to see that "everything is connected to everything else by a Presence whose power is infinite, exquisitely gentle, yet rock solid."

Great works of art, music and literature are written by individuals who have transcended the level of Peace, and these are the works that are both sublime and timeless, according to Dr. Hawkins. The works produced by these individuals actually have the power to lift others temporarily into higher levels of consciousness, he says.

The enlightenment level is reached only by a very few and is akin to a level close to mankind's definition of divinity, according to Dr. Hawkins. Citing Krishna and Buddha as examples, he explains in his book that "This is the level of powerful inspiration; these beings set in place attractor energy fields that influence all mankind."

According to Dr. Hawkins's book, about "85 percent of the human race calibrates below the critical level of 200." The collective conscious of the human race is only about 207, he maintains. About four percent of the human population has an energy field above 500, only 0.4 are above 540, and only one in ten million exceeds level 600.

Given those statistics, it is immediately evident that progressing from one level to another is not easy. The energy it takes to move between levels is what gave rise to the title of Dr. Hawkins' book, "Power vs. Force." Dr. Hawkins maintains that the power of force must constantly be fed. Force pulls people down. Elements of force, according to Dr. Harris, include judgment, which is destructive. Power lifts people up away from

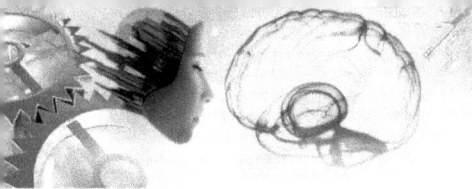

the energy of force. Elements of power, like compassion, give life and energy.

To lift one out from the negative power of force and progress from one level to the next requires help from others. Unless they engage the power of greater attractor forces, Hawkins says, people will continue to fight against the external circumstances and lower attraction forces and be pulled down by them.

There are natural progressions to each level, and it is necessary to master things in one level before one is able to be successful in the next.

Steve Pavlina puts it this way on Stevepavlina.com:

"Going up even one level can be extremely hard; most people don't do so in their entire lives. A change in just one level can radically alter everything in your life.

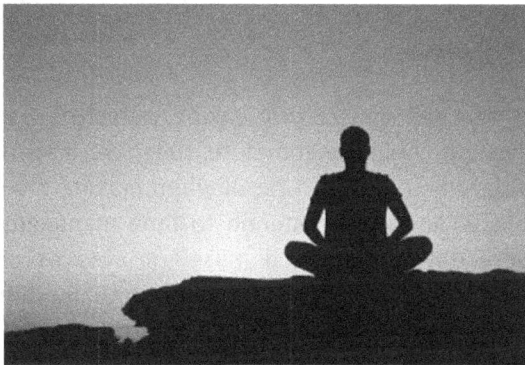

This is why people below the level of courage aren't likely to progress without external help. Courage is required to work on this consciously; it comes down to repeatedly betting your whole reality for the chance to become more conscious and

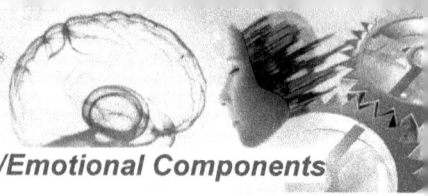

aware. However, whenever you reach that next level, you realize clearly that it was a good bet. For example, when you hit the level of courage, all your past fears and false pride seem silly to you now. When you reach the level of acceptance (setting and achieving goals), you look back on the level of willingness and see you were like a mouse running on a treadmill — you were a good runner, but you didn't pick a direction (Steve Pavlina, 2012)."

Dr. Hawkins maintains that 85 percent of all human beings live below the Courage level. The positive power that would be created by individuals transcending just one level would be significant, he believes. Still, Dr. Hawkins believes that statistically, the average person advances about five points over an entire lifetime. Because of these factors, and others, Dr. Hawkins writes in his book that 2.6 percent of the entire population accounts for 76 percent of the world's problems. Societal change, he asserts, will only happen as individuals begin to reach for, and find, higher attractor patterns.

Steve Pavlina writes:

"We have to keep consciously taking ourselves back to the sources that can help us complete the next leap. Each step requires different solutions. I recall when making the shift from neutrality to willingness, I listened to time management tapes almost every day. I immersed myself in sources created by people at the level of willingness until I eventually shifted. But a book on time management will be of little use to someone who's at the level of pride; they'll reject the very notion with a lot of defensiveness. And time management is meaningless to someone at the level of peace. But you can't hit the higher levels if you haven't mastered the basics first. . . . We all have to start somewhere."

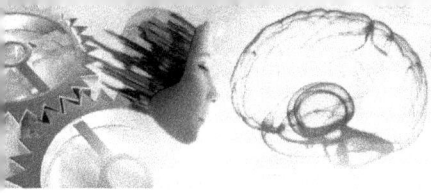

Dr. Hawkins maintains that just treating society will not bring about lasting change. He notes that there is a difference between treating and healing. Legislation, market changes, and even war are not permanent solutions. Societies have seen all these remedies and serious problems continue to occur. Permanent change will only happen with real healing, which involves employing positive attractors like unconditional kindness and compassion, he writes.

Vibrational Healing

The idea of vibrational medicine has developed in the wake of Dr. Hawkins's findings. The foundation of vibrational medicine is the idea that all matter on earth, both living and non-living, vibrates on a definite, measurable frequency. The theory proposes that the frequency changes according to our individual level of consciousness.

The idea of vibrational healing, also called Energy Healing, proposes that because all matter emits a frequency, that frequency can be used to heal by restoring it to the proper balance. Vibrational Medicine inherently promotes the idea that good health flows from the appropriate balance of energy, while things that disrupt that flow lead to illness. For hundreds of years, western mystics and spiritualists from India and the Far East have held that poor health habits and negative emotions are the basis for many illnesses.

Prana, a spiritual tradition of India, Ch'i in China, and even many of the traditions of the Native Americans have had energy healing as their basis. Modern holographic patterning, Kirlian photography, and cutting edge methods of energy scanning have developed information about the human energy field.

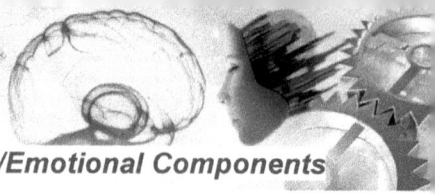

These scientific studies have created new ways to promote vibrational health.

Vibration is often likened to frequency. Scientists have long known that different frequencies reflect different patterns of vibration. If Dr. Hawkins is correct, then reconfiguring the vibration, or life energy pattern, of an individual will bring health and vitality.

The human energy field is called the "aura". Medieval paintings of the Saints often depict this aura as a halo. Scientists have long known that humans have this energy field. It moves with the body. For example, if a person extends their arms, the aura moves with their arms. Scientists and mystics propose that energy is light, and humans are beings of light. However, a limited sense of the world prevents people from consciously perceiving the subtle energy fields in the surroundings.

The Japanese practice of Reiki, developed by Japanese Buddhist Mikao Usui, is based on the idea that a transfer and balance of energy is possible. Reiki is a practice of laying hands on a person to transfer the energy from an external force, which some call a God force. Some say that the power of Reiki is nearly miraculous. Reiki is used to treat people who are under emotional, physical, or mental stress. Reiki is also said to be a viable support to other, more traditional, methods of treatment.

Quantum Touch, or QT, is another accepted form of vibrational healing. It is based on the understanding that every human has an energy field that can be of assistance to another person. Quantum Touch combines breathing and energy awareness techniques to transfer life-force energy in a way that is targeted and strengthened.

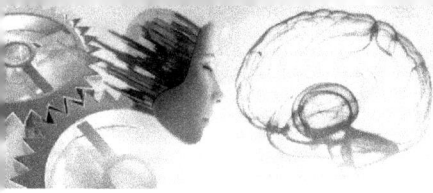

Similar to polarity therapy, which seeks to balance opposite energy poles, Quantum Touch is touted as a way to focus light energy to improve a person's well being. Some say that QT also has caused the proper alignment of the body's bones to occur spontaneously. Advanced Quantum Touch methods often employ the spinning of the chakras or harmonic toning as well.

Many health care facilities now allow or even invite therapists that practice Reiki, Polarity, or Quantum Touch. Modern medicine has long relied on medicinal and surgical treatments. As studies are done, many physicians today are open to alternative treatments.

Vibrational or energy healing are not limited to Reiki, Polarity, and Quantum Touch, however. Advances in homeopathy, aromatherapy, acupuncture, chiropractic treatment and other energy-adjusting therapies are also gaining acceptance. The basis for all of these types of vibrational therapies is that any illness requires the treatment of the whole person.

Energy Therapy seeks to revitalize the entire person, causing "stuck" energy to flow freely again. As energy flows, the resulting purification process begins to heal the illness and its underlying psychic cause. This restored balance of energy brings new health, balance and mental and spiritual vitality.

A few chiropractic physicians who are highly trained in energy, vibration, frequency medicine and techniques can raise levels of consciousness and levels of super-consciousness. This process may take anywhere between one minute to an hour, depending on the patient/individual and can only be done by a highly trained practitioner. These techniques allow the raising of level of consciousness at a more rapid rate, accomplishing high levels of maturity, wisdom and enlightenment.

Scientists have long understood that there are at least two basic levels of consciousness – the conscious and the subconscious mind. As studies evolve, many have come to believe that there is a third primary level, the superconscious mind.

The conscious mind is that part of a person that is acutely aware of what is going on around them. It is the part of the mind used for thinking, planning, learning, and imagining. The subconscious mind lies deep within the brain and is the place where dreams, memories, emotions, and beliefs dwell. The elements of the subconscious mind have great power over the actions of the conscious mind.

The super conscious mind is suspected of being the part of a person that connects with the intuitive and spiritual realm. Many suspect that this part of the mind may be the most powerful.

As science advances, it is becoming clear that the universe is powered by wave energy. Quantum physics has proposed that these energy waves represent some form of higher intelligence. Measuring the physical vibrations of matter is only beginning to reveal the power inherent in those energy fields.

From ancient times, people have known that there is energy outside of what they could see. Premonition and intuition have been powerful forces throughout history. The study of universal energy fields is only growing, as the limits of modern medicine are becoming known. Physicians, mystics, spiritual healers, and others are becoming united in the realization that there is a force in nature that can be harnessed for great good.

The power of an energy-transforming touch to bring emotional, spiritual, and physical healing cannot be underestimated. As more is learned about the balance of energy and how it affects

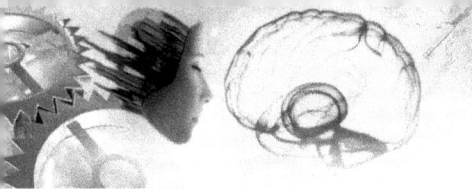

everything from an individual cell to an entire society, mankind will only benefit. As more is learned about the many levels of consciousness, more will be learned about how to bring perfect balance and growth to individuals and the world around them.

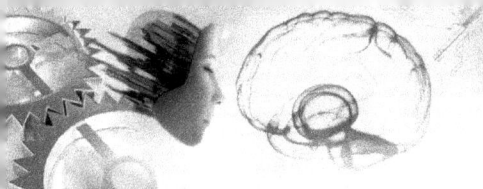

Bibliography

Chapter 1:

Health Triangle. (n.d.). *Coach Splendorio's Health Class*. Retrieved May 16, 2012, from http://oreoj12.tripod.com/id14.html

Benefits of Chiropractic Care - Grosse Pointe Woods Chiropractor - Triangle Chiropractic and Massage - Chiropractors in Grosse Pointe Woods, MI. (n.d.). *Chiropractor - Triangle Chiropractic and Massage - Chiropractors in Grosse Pointe Woods, MI*. Retrieved May 16, 2012, from
http://www.drtsakos.com/library/3920/BenefitsofChiropracticCare.ht ml

Applied Kinesiology Clinic. (n.d.). *Applied Kinesology Clinic*. Retrieved May 16, 2012, from http://www.appliedkinesiologyclinic.com/net_intro_pg2.htm

Improving Emotional Health: Strategies and Tips for Good Mental Health. (n.d.). *Helpguide helps you help yourself to better mental and emotional health*. Retrieved May 16, 2012, from http://www.helpguide.org/mental/mental_emotional_health.htm

Burton, D. B., DC., CCN., PA., & Physician, a. C. (n.d.). The Triad of Health. *Chiropractic Physician, Clinical Nutritionist, and Acupuncturist in Plantation,Florida*. Retrieved May 16, 2012, from http://www.betterbacks.com/triad.htm

Chapter 2:

Hans Selye (1956); The Stress of Life, New York: McGraw-Hill, Koolhaas, J., et al. (2011); "Stress revisited: A critical evaluation of the stress concept." Neuroscience and Biobehavioral Reviews 35

Kemeny, M. E. (2007). "Understanding the interaction between psychosocial stress and immune-related diseases: A stepwise progression." Brain, Behavior, and Immunity

Lazarus, R.S. (1966). Psychological Stress and the Coping Process; New York: McGraw-Hill.

Melucci, N. (2004). Psychology; Barron's Educational Series, Hauppauge, NY

Allen R. (1983); Human stress: its nature and control; Burgess press; Minneapolis

Amen. D. (1998); Change your brain, Change your life; Three Rivers Press; New York

Everly G, Rosenfeld R. (1981) The nature and treatment of stress response; Plenum Press; New York

McEwen B. (2002) The end of stress as we know it; Joseph Henry Press; Washington DC

Chapter 3:

Emotion in Psychology 101 at AllPsych Online. (n.d.). *Psychology Classroom at AllPsych Online*. Retrieved May 15, 2012, from http://allpsych.com/psychology101/emotion.html

Theories about emotion. (n.d.). *Changing minds and persuasion -- How we change what others think, believe, feel and do*. Retrieved May 15, 2012, from http://changingminds.org/explanations/theories/a_emotion.htm

Infinite Minds - Learning 2.0 - Understanding Brainwaves and Mental States. (n.d.). *Infinite Minds : Discover your Potential*. Retrieved May 15, 2012, from http://infiniteminds.info/Learning-2.0/Brainwave-Entrainment/Understanding-Brainwaves-and-Mental-States.html

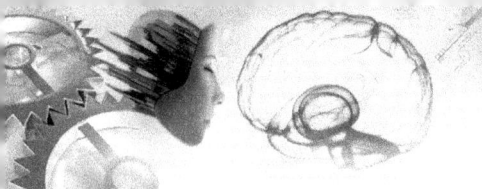

Chiropractic And The Emotions. (n.d.). *Australasian Home of Torque Release Technique*. Retrieved May 15, 2012, from http://www.torquerelease.com.au/Mind-Body.htm

Heartburn Home Remedies: Herbs & Other Natural Remedies. (n.d.). *WebMD - Better information. Better health.*. Retrieved May 15, 2012, from http://www.webmd.com/heartburn-gerd/home-heartburn-remedies-natural-remedies-heartburn

DeAngelis, T. (n.d.). One treatment for emotional disorders?. *American Psychological Association (APA)*. Retrieved May 15, 2012, from http://www.apa.org/monitor/2008/10/disorders.aspx

Our emotional health intelligence emotion. (n.d.). *our emotional health intelligence emotion*. Retrieved May 15, 2012, from http://www.our-emotional-health.com/

Chapter 4:

Philosophy 156: Different Kinds of Mental States. (n.d.). *Jim Pryor*. Retrieved May 15, 2012, from http://www.jimpryor.net/teaching/courses/mind/notes/mentalstates.html

Mental States. (n.d.). *Mental States*. Retrieved May 15, 2012, from http://www.mentalstates.net/

Identifying mental states from neural states under mental constraints . (n.d.). *Interface Focus* . Retrieved May 15, 2012, from http://rsfs.royalsocietypublishing.org/content/2/1/74.short

Infinite Minds - Learning 2.0 - Understanding Brainwaves and Mental States. (n.d.). *Infinite Minds : Discover your Potential*. Retrieved May 15, 2012, from http://infiniteminds.info/Learning-2.0/Brainwave-Entrainment/Understanding-Brainwaves-and-Mental-States.html

Chiropractic in Mental Ailments. (n.d.). *Old And Sold Antiques Auction*. Retrieved May 15, 2012, from http://www.oldandsold.com/articles09/chiropractic-14.shtml

Chapter 5:

The difference between rest and sleep. (n.d.). *sleep problems* . Retrieved May 15, 2012, from http://www.help-with-sleep-problems.com/rest-and-sleep.html

Snoring and Sleep Apnea | AAOMS.org. (n.d.). *American Association of Oral and Maxillofacial Surgeons (AAOMS)*. Retrieved May 15, 2012, from http://www.aaoms.org/sleep_apnea.php

Relief From Sleep Disorders by American Chiropractic, Providing Chiropractic Care in Louisville, Kentucky (KY). (n.d.). *Contact American Chiropractic in Louisville, Kentucky (KY)*. Retrieved May 15, 2012, from http://www.adjustmenow.com/sleep.htm

5 Ways To Evaluate "Alternative Medicines" | The Consumer Warning Network. (n.d.). *The Consumer Warning Network*. Retrieved May 15, 2012, from http://www.consumerwarningnetwork.com/2008/12/30/5-ways-to-evaluate-alternative-medicines/

Melatonin and Sleep | National Sleep Foundation - Information on Sleep Health and Safety. (n.d.). *National Sleep Foundation - Information on Sleep Health and Safety | Information on Sleep Health and Safety*. Retrieved May 15, 2012, from http://www.sleepfoundation.org/article/sleep-topics/melatonin-and-sleep

Herbal medicine. (n.d.). *University of Maryland Medical Center | Home*. Retrieved May 15, 2012, from http://www.umm.edu/altmed/articles/herbal-medicine-000351.htm

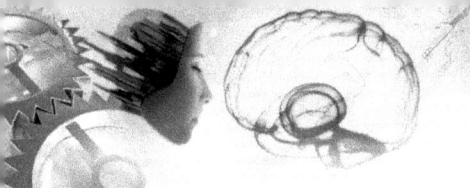

Chapter 6:

Levels of Consciousness. (n.d.). *Personal Development for Smart People - Steve Pavlina*. Retrieved May 15, 2012, from http://www.stevepavlina.com/blog/2005/04/levels-of-consciousness/

obtunded., First, m. c., coma, o. d., & steps., t. (n.d.). Level of Consciousness - Clinical Methods - NCBI Bookshelf. *National Center for Biotechnology Information*. Retrieved May 15, 2012, from http://www.ncbi.nlm.nih.gov/books/NBK380/

12 Stages of Healing. (n.d.). *Network Chiropractic and CranioSacral Therapy*. Retrieved May 15, 2012, from http://www.10ac.com/12stages.htm

Infinite Minds - Learning 2.0 - Understanding Brainwaves and Mental States. (n.d.). *Infinite Minds : Discover your Potential*. Retrieved May 15, 2012, from http://infiniteminds.info/Learning-2.0/Brainwave-Entrainment/Understanding-Brainwaves-and-Mental-States.html

Consciousness Defined. (n.d.). *Speed of Light Films*. Retrieved May 15, 2012, from http://speedoflightfilms.com/index.php/consciousness.html

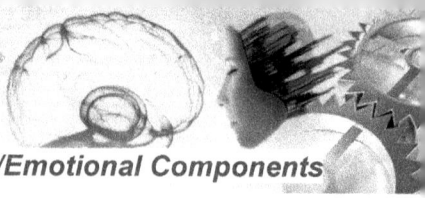

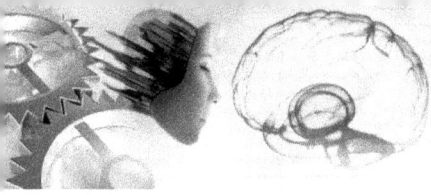

Picture Credits:

The publisher would like to thank the following for their kind permission to reproduce their photographs:

Wikimedia Commons for public Domain Images used in various chapters of this book.

Also, more specifically, the various images below were reproduced with the permission of their respective creators:

Chapter 1:

lossy-page1-442px-Brain_Microvessel by Nathan S. Ivey.tif

Chapter 2:

415px-Tension-headache by Shanghai killer whale

1129px-Cholesterol_Spacefill by RedAndr

Chapter 3:

Strong_emotion by Arwen Abendstem

Paleo_food by trmdttr

800px-Herbs_for_sabzi_polo by tannaz from los angeles

Chapter 5:

800px-Sleeping_the_day_away_-_3087394718 by Pedro Simões from Lisboa, Portugal

Chapter 6:

401px-Falun_Gong_adherents_meditating from http://hqphoto.minghui.org/photo_high/allimages/Pict0006.jpg

All the remaining images in the book are from:

FreeDigitalPhotos.net

About the Author

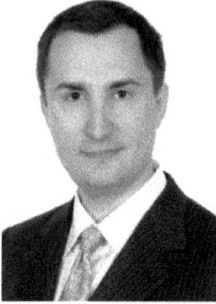

Dr. Vladimir Gordin is a man who needs no introduction. He has been a leading practitioner of Chiropractic and of the healing arts for over a decade. Using methods that show his innate understanding of the human organism, Dr. Gordin has changed the lives of thousands of patients. Dr. Gordin also lectures regularly on health related issues, and has his own highly popular radio show listened to in over 20 countries on five continents.

Dr. Gordin's qualifications include his Doctorate in Chiropractic from the prestigious National University of Health Sciences, his degrees in Biology and Physics and Human Biology, and post-graduate studies that have qualified him to be Board Eligible Diplomate in Chiropractic Orthopedics and Applied Kinesiology, as well as Board Candidate Diplomate in Clinical Nutrition. He also holds certifications that grant him mastery over a large variety of treatment protocols. His qualifications and considerable experience allow Dr. Gordin to use a vast array of highly effective methods and techniques.

*The **core** of Dr. Gordin's **philosophy** is treating the root cause of a patient's problems. His **goal** is to help his patients towards lasting and permanent health, guiding them towards a gentle, yet rapid, recovery.*

This series of books by Dr. Gordin is an expression of this philosophy and goal...

Dr. Gordin resides with his beautiful wife and three children in Chicago, IL.

www.ingramcontent.com/pod-product-compliance
Lightning Source LLC
Chambersburg PA
CBHW071133280326
41935CB00010B/1215